AF413303

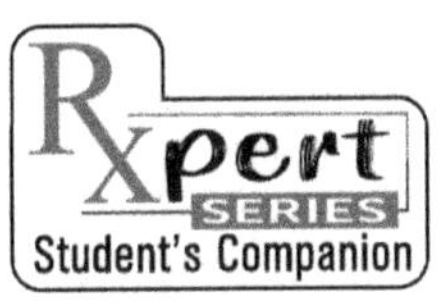

Quick Review on

Herbal Drug Technology

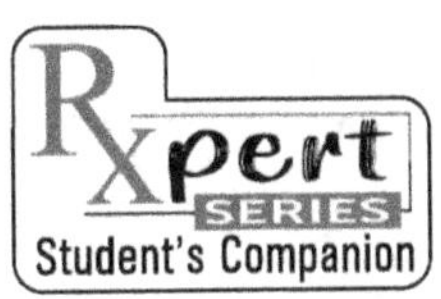

Quick Review on

Herbal Drug Technology

Dr. Vivekananda Mandal

[Former WERC Researcher, Govt. of Japan]
Assistant Professor
Division of Pharmacognosy
Department of Pharmacy
Guru Ghasidas Vishwavidyalaya
(A Central University)
Bilaspur (C.G) 495009, India

Mr. Kavi Bhushan Singh Chouhan
Senior Research Fellow
Division of Pharmacognosy
Department of Pharmacy
Guru Ghasidas Vishwavidyalaya
(A Central University)
Bilaspur (C.G) 495009, India

Dr. Roshni Tandey
Assistant Professor
Department of Pharmacognosy
Apollo College of Pharmacy
Durg (C.G), India

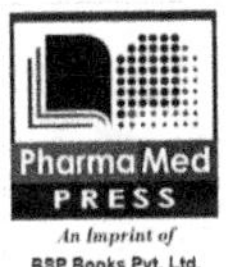

PharmaMed Press

An imprint of BSP Books pvt. Ltd
4-4-309/316, Giriraj Lane,
Sultan Bazar, Hyderabad - 500 095.

Quick Review on Herbal Drug Technology
by Vivekananda Mandal, Kavi Bhushan Singh Chouhan and Roshni Tandey

© 2023, by Publisher

Published by:

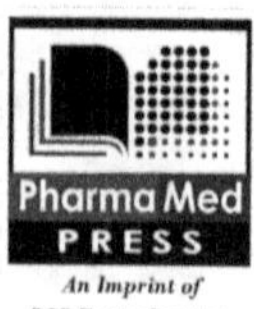

PharmaMed Press
An imprint of BSP Books Pvt. Ltd.
4-4-309/316, Giriraj Lane, Sultan Bazar, Hyderabad - 500 095.
Phone: 040-23445688; Fax: 91+40-23445611
e-mail: info@pharmamedpress.com
www.pharmamedpress.com/pharmamedpress.net

ISBN: 978-93-91910-22-8 (Hardback)

Preface

The book's foundation was laid during the tough times of COVID pandemic induced lockdown periods. In such a tough time, considering the academic needs of the students and in order to facilitate their exam preparation, it was decided to hand over to them an exam companion in the form of a book. This book shall refresh the students' thought processes and help them configure their preparation according to the exam requirements. The book covers the entire PCI prescribed syllabus in questions and answers (two marks, five marks and ten marks). Thus, the book shall serve as an exhaustive question bank and shall provide an extra edge to the students in their exam preparation. Scoring in the examination needs strategic preparation and the book is expected to provide the same. The answers have been drafted in simple language in order to make them compatible with students thought process. The book shall ease the exam stress and serve as a one-stop destination for examinees who now need not burn their midnight oil for exam preparation.

The authors would like to thank their family members who were pillars of support and strength during this pandemic. The authors would also like to thank the frontline Corona Warriors, whose tiresome efforts helped us to combat the virus. The authors would like to wish all the students a happy, healthy and smart exam preparation, and the book shall be your best companion in this regard.

- Authors

Contents

Herbs as Raw Materials, Biodynamic Agriculture, Indian Systems of Medicine

Two marks category questions

1. Define herbs?

Herbs include crude leafy green flowering plants, which areshort-lived and do not have a woody stem. It could be either perennial, biennial, or annual in nature. Such plants generally have aromatic properties, are sometimes used as food, and may also possess medicinal properties. Vegetables do not constitute herbs. Any plant part, namely leaves, stems, flowers, fruit, stem, bark, roots, rhizomes, or even the entire plant, preferably in an unprocessed manner, can be called a herb. Example – Tulsi.

2. Define Herbal medicine?

Includes herbs, herbal materials, herbal preparations, and finished herbal products.

3. Define herbal material?

Whole or fragmented plant parts (leaves, roots, bark, rhizomes, etc.) in an unprocessed state generally in dried form.They include herbs, fresh juices, gums, fixed oils, essential oils, resins, and dry powders of herbs.

4. Define herbal drugs?

Herbal drugs are also known as herbal substances and indicate the part of the plant which is used for therapeutic purposes. Such plant parts can be in the form of a whole plant or any specific part (like leaves, roots, barks, etc.). These parts may be available in cut, fragmented, or even powdered forms obtained from both higher plants (like turmeric, neem) as well as lower plants (like algae, fungi, etc.).

5. Define herbal medicinal products?

Any medicinal product is specifically exhibiting its therapeutic effect due to the presence of single or multiple herbal drugs or various herbal drug preparations or a combination of both herbal drugs and herbal preparations: for example – Brahmi capsules.

6. What do you mean by herbal drug preparation?

Outcome or final end product obtained after subjecting herbal drugs either in crude form or processed form to different extraction methods (like maceration, Soxhlet extraction, distillation, expression, etc.) and other methods such as purification, enrichment, or fermentation. Example- extract obtained after maceration, essential oil obtained after distillation, juices obtained after expression.

7. What do you mean by herbal remedy?

Usage of herbal products for therapeutic purposes is known as a herbal remedy. For example, the use of various herbal products for the management of diabetes and herbal products for the management of COVID-19 infection is a good example of herbal remedy where certain herbal products are used to treat or manage a particular disease. The herbal remedy may also come under the drug regulations in a specific country.

8. What do you mean by herbal teas?

Herbal teas are aqueous decoctions or infusions prepared from a single herbal drug or a mixture of herbal drugs for oral consumption. It is one type of herbal preparation which the end-user prepares just before consumption.

9. Define markers.

Markers indicate chemically defined specific phytoconstituents or any group of phytoconstituents present in a herbal drug and which can be qualitatively and quantitatively used for determining the quality of the drug and finished product as well. The presence of the minimum quantity of the marker is essential for declaring the crude drug or finished product as fit in terms of quality for further use. If the crude drug is found to contain the desired quantity of the marker,then it can be further used for processing of finished products, and if the finished product is found to contain the desired quantity of the marker, it can be considered fit for human use.

a) Analytical markers – such markers do not have therapeutic value, but their quantity determines the quality of the crude drug or finished herbal product. They are used mainly for analytical purposes.

b) Active markers or bio-markers – such markers have biological activity and play a vital role in thestandardization of medicinal plants and herbal products. The presence of a minimum quantity of the desired biomarker ensures the exhibition of the intended biological effect by the crude drug or herbal product. For example – curcumin is the marker for turmeric. So, in order to declare turmeric rhizomes fit for use, they must contain the specified amount of curcumin. If a finished herbal product containing turmeric is to be used, in order to pass the quality test and to ensure that the final product will exhibit the desired medicinal effect, the final product should contain the desired quantity of curcumin.

10. List out the sources of herbs.

The different sources of herbs are,

a) Plants: Includes both higher plants (angiosperms and gymnosperms) and lower plants like algae, fungi, lichens, and bryophytes (mosses and liverworts). Example – Higher plants: leaves (tulsi), flowers (clove bud), fruits (amla), roots (rauwolfia), rhizomes (podophyllum, ginger), lower plants: ergot, algae

b) Marine sources: Organisms found in the marine ecosystem which serve as excellent drug sources are sponges, tunicates, fishes, soft corals, sea hares, mollusks, echinoderms, bryozoans, prawns, shells, sea slugs, marine microorganisms, and phytoplankton's. Such aquatic living organisms have been screened for antibacterial, cardioactive, immunomodulator, anti-fungal, anti-inflammatory, anticancer, antimicrobial, neuroprotective, analgesic, toxins, and antimalarial properties. Examples of clinically approved marine drugs: - Cytarabine (used in leukemia), Vidarabine (used in recurrent epithelial keratitis caused by HSV), Ziconotide (analgesic), and Trabectedin (used for the treatment of ovarian cancer).

c) Plant tissue culture: It is an artificial method of growing plants (*in-vitro* multiplication of plant cells) in laboratory conditions on a defined solid or liquid medium under aseptic conditions through various biotechnological interventions. Example – production of catharanthine from *Catharanthus roseus*, Diosgenin from *Dioscorea doryphore*, reserpine from *Rauwolfia* species, Ginsenosides from *Panax ginseng* are some good examples of drugs obtained through the tissue culture method.

11. What is the basis of the selection of herbal materials for research purposes?

Herbal materials (plant parts) are selected for research purposes based on the following criteria's,

a) Ethnobotanical data: herbal material can be selected based on their ethnic use or existing use in society. Such herbal materials, if in use among a particular community for several generations, then the drug discovery research from such plant materials is likely to yield sure success.

b) Chemotaxonomy data: based on chemotaxonomic relations, plants can be selected for research. Plants belonging to a particular family share some common phytoconstituents. Hence, if the plant family is identified by a taxonomist, a judicious decision regarding the probable presence of particular chemical constituents and possible use of the plant can be made. Example – Solanaceae family are rich in tropane alkaloids.

c) Random selection: plants are selected based on random phytochemical screening and high throughput screening based on *in-vitro* enzyme assay methods. Plants responding positively to the presence of some phytoconstituents through *in-vitro* enzyme-substrate assay methods are further taken up for lab-based research. Chances of success in ending up with a drug-like compound are fewer.

d) Traditional information-based approach: information obtained from traditional systems of medicine such as Ayurveda, Unani can form the basis of plant selection. Such plants which are extensively used in traditional systems of medicine are likely to yield success in drug discovery research.

e) Zoo-pharmacognosy approach: close monitoring and observation of grazing and wild animals can provide vital leads in search of herbs for research purposes with special reference to drug discovery.

12. Explain the selection criteria of herbal materials for inclusion in WHO monographs

There are two major criteria for the selection of herbal material for its inclusion in WHO monographs which are as follows,

a) Must be in common use in any two WHO regions

b) Availability of sufficient scientific data to satisfy monograph data requirements. Example – data on purity tests (microbiological, chemical, heavy metal, radioactive contamination data), chemical assays, and pharmacological activity must be available as per requirement for establishing a monograph.

13. What is the significance of proper identification and authentication of herbal materials in herbal drug manufacturing?

Medicinal plants (herbal materials) are the starting material in medicinal plant research or herbal drug manufacturing. Henceforth, a wrong identification or a non-judicious selection of any herbal material is sufficient enough to spoil the latter stages to come, thus compromising the entire objective. Herbal materials are valued because of the medicinal activity of the phytoconstituents present in them, whose quantity determines the quality of the finished product. Proper identification and authentication,which ensures quality, safety, and efficacy of herbal medicine, are important because of the following reasons,

a) Adulteration: in order to ensure that herbal materials are free from any kind of adulteration (intentional or unintentional).

b) Correct species: in order to ensure that taxonomically correct species have been selected.

c) Quality: in order to ensure that substandard herbal materials are not used as starting material. Quality is determined by ensuring that the desired phytoconstituents are present in the right quantity enough for exhibiting the desired pharmacological activity.

d) To counter variability in the quality of herbal raw material due to geographical differences associated with its cultivation.

14. **Name the different methods employed in making herbal preparations.**

Herbal preparations are made by subjecting the herbal raw materials (either processed or unprocessed), usually in dried form, to methods like maceration, Soxhlet extraction, percolation, infusion, decoction, digestion, distillation (herbal materials are used in fresh form for extraction of essential oil), microwave-assisted extraction, supercritical fluid extraction (for extraction of essential oil) and fractionation techniques for purification purposes. Such herbal preparations can be used directly for therapeutic purposes if prepared under GMP conditions or may be used as intermediates for making the finished herbal medicinal product or various other herbal dosage forms.

15. **List out and define the constant parameters involved in quantitative microscopy for quality control of herbal raw material.**

a) Stomatal Index: Stomatal index is defined as the percentage ratio of the number of stomata to the total number of epidermal cells. The stomatal number may vary with the age of the leaf species, but the stomatal index is relatively constant for a given species.

Stomatal Index $= S \times 100 \div (E + S)$

S = number of stomata in a given area of the leaf surface

E = number of epidermal cell in the same area

b) Palisade ratio: it is defined as the average number of palisade cells beneath each epidermal cell, using four continuous epidermal cells for the count. It is determined with the help of camera lucida.

c) Vein-Islet number: the mesophyll tissue of a leaf is divided into small portions of photosynthetic tissues by the branching of veins and veinlets. These small portions so formed midway between midrib and margin of the leaf are known as vein-islet. The number of such vein-islets per sq. mm of the leaf surface is known as the vein-islet number. The value is constant for a leaf species unaffected by the age or size of the leaf. Useful parameter for identifying closely related species.

d) Vein-Termination number: it is defined as the number of veinlet termination per mm^2 of the leaf surface. The value is constant for a leaf species unaffected by the age or size of the leaf. Useful parameter for identifying closely related species.

The above parameters are constant for a given leaf species, and doesn't change with the age or size of the leaf. Collectively they are known as leaf constants, and such data obtained from test samples can be matched with reference data provided in official books for identification and authentication of the correct plant species. It is a very useful tool for quality control in the case of powdered drugs.

16. What do you mean by stomatal number? Mention the functions of stomata.

It is defined as the average number of stomata present per mm^2 of the leaf surface. Stomata help in gaseous exchange (respiration) and transpiration.

17. What do you mean by pest and pest management?

Pests are those species of plants and animals which are undesirable to humans and can potentially reduce the availability, quality, and value of any human resource like agricultural crops.

Pests are natural invaders for any agricultural products and can cause huge damage to crops if not controlled. Pests includes weeds (unwanted invasive plants), certain bacteria, fungi (*Phytophthora nicotianae*) and viruses (Mosaic viruses), rodents (rats), nematodes, mites, and various plant feeding insects (locusts, grasshoppers). Pest management involves all those procedures adopted to reduce the number of pests in any agricultural production to an acceptable threshold by using various biological, chemical, physical, and genetic methods.

18. What do you mean by integrated pest management?

Integrated pest management is a long-term approach that focuses on developing an ecosystem committed towards long-term prevention of damage occurring through pests by achieving effective optimal integration of various methods such as biological control, habitat alteration, changes in agricultural practices, and use of various pest-resistant species.

19. What do you mean by crop rotation? Give its significance.

Crop rotation is the practice of growing different crops sequentially in the same land (plot) in different seasons. It helps in optimizing soil nutrients, improves soil fertility, and helps in eradicating pests and weeds.

20. Name the various disciplines of Ayurveda.

Ayurveda has eight disciplines collectively known as 'Ashtanga Ayurveda'. They are as follows,

- Kayachikitsa (internal medicine)
- Bhootavidya (treating psychological diseases)
- Kaumar Bhritya (pediatric)
- Rasayana (treating geriatric patients)
- Vajikarna (use of aphrodisiacs)
- Shalya (surgery)
- Shalakya (eye and ear)
- Agada tantra (toxins related)

21. Name some ancient Indian medicinal manuscripts.

Rig-Veda, Yajur-Veda, Atharva-Veda, Dhanwantari Nighantu, Charak Samhita and Sushruta Samhita.

22. Name the seven standards of the human body as per the Unani System.

The seven standards of the human body are Mizaj (temperaments), Anza (organs), Quo (resources), Arkan (components), Arawh (spirits), Aklath (humours), and Afal (capacities).

23. Differentiate between Ayurveda and Siddha systems of medicine.

	Ayurveda	Siddha
1.	Prevalent throughout India	Prevalent more in Tamil culture
2.	Initially practiced by saints	Initially practiced by Siddhars
3.	Ayurvedic formulations consist of medicinal plants	Formulations mainly consist of metals and minerals
4.	Involves concept of Panchamahabhutas and Triodosha	Apart from Panchamahabhutas and Tridosha also involves concept of Siva and Sakthi
5.	Pancha karma mode of therapy is used	Ashtasthana Pareeksha mode of therapy
6.	Premier institute of Ayurveda = National institute of Ayurveda, Jaipur	Premier institute of Siddha = National institute of Siddha, Chennai
7.	Practioner of Ayurveda is known as Vaidya or Vaidyaraja	Practioner are known as Siddhars
8.	Charaka was one of the principal contributors of Ayurveda	Agasthava is belived to be the founder father of Siddha

24. What are the advantages of the fermentation process used inthe preparation of Asavas-Arishtas.

a) Removes sugars from the plant material and improves bioavailability

b) Provides better extraction efficiency due to gradually rising alcohol strength during the fermentation process

c) Yeast cells act as cleansing agents by binding with heavy metals and pesticides

d) Neutralizesthe toxic effects of some phytoconstituents

e) Fermentation ruptures the plant cells and exposes them to the bacteria and enzymes for necessary transformation.

25. What is the difference between asavas and arishtas.

	Asavas	Arishtas
1.	Fresh or dried crude drug is used	Dried crude drug is used
2.	If fresh crude drug is used – juice is extracted by expression If dried crude drug is used – infusion is prepared	Decoction of the crude drug is the starting material
3.	No heat is used for preparing the starting material which is either juice or infusion	Heat is used for preparation of decoction

26. What do you mean by 'churna'?

Churna is an ayurvedic formulation consisting of a single or mixture of crude drugs in fine free-flowing powder form in a dry state. Desired plants are cleaned, dried, powdered, and passed through sieve#80 to obtain very fine homogenous particles. Lesser is the particle size, greater shall be the surface area resulting in better absorption from GIT. They can be consumed along with water, milk, honey, or ghee. Churna's are also converted into pills or tablets for proper dosing. The efficacy of churna may be influenced by the time of intake, like whether it is consumed before or after a meal. They are mostly used for the treatment of constipation, indigestion, and diabetes. Example – Triphala churna, Trikatu churna, ashwagandha churna, etc.

27. What do you mean by Gutika?

Gutika is an ayurvedic preparation where a single or a mixture of powdered drugs are cooked with jaggery or macerated with honey to achieve a thick consistency and rolled into circular-shaped pills. When the same consistency is rolled in the shape of an elongated table like, it is known as Vatika.

28. Mention the constituents of the final reaction mixture, which is made to undergo fermentation for the preparation of arishta and asava.

For asavas: juice extracted from fresh crude drug or infusion prepared from dried crude drug + jaggery or honey (fermentation medium) + flavouring agent + additional powdered drug (if any) + powdered flower of *Woodfordia fruticosa* (source of yeast to initiate fermentation).

For arishta: decoction of crude drug + jaggery or honey (fermentation medium) + flavouring agent + powdered flower of *Woodfordia fruticosa* (source of yeast to initiate fermentation).

29. What is Kashaya?

It is an ayurvedic preparation basically consisting of an aqueous extract of the crude drug.

30. Mention the various types of ayurvedic formulations.

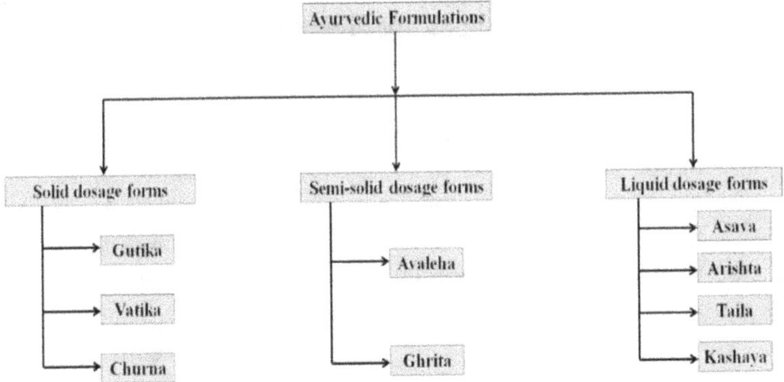

Five marks category questions

31. List out and explain the different sources of crude drugs.
Herbs can be obtained from different sources, which have been explained below,

d) **Plant source:** refers to terrestrial plants (both higher and lower plants). Herbs can be obtained from seed-bearing plants such as angiosperms (flowering plants) and gymnosperms (non-flowering plants). Angiosperms are a good source of plants rich in glycosides and essential oils. Gymnosperms predominantly contain constituents such as alkaloids (example –ergot alkaloids in ephedra). Both the typesof plants have profound use in folk and traditional medicine and their different parts such as leaves (senna), flowers (clove buds), seeds (nux-vomica, nutmeg), fruits (amla), bark (cinchona), roots (podophyllum) and rhizomes (turmeric) are frequently used for medicinal purposes. The other type is lower plants, whichincludealgae, fungi, lichens, and bryophytes (mosses and liverworts). Among lower plants, microscopic and macroscopic algae have been predominantly used as a source for antioxidant, anticancer, and antiviral compounds.

e) **Marine sources**: Marine environment provides a unique natural habitat, and the living organisms available in the marine environment are totally different from those available in the terrestrial environment. The marine environment is very challenging because of the very drastic conditions prevailing inside the ocean with the continuous threat from changing oceanic environment and various predators. In the process to survive such drastic living conditions, marine organisms continually evolve themselves by producing various biochemicals which help them to adapt to the marine ecosystem. Such chemicals, if scientifically explored, could be beneficial to humans. Organisms found in the marine ecosystem and which serve as excellent drug sources are sponges, tunicates, fishes, soft corals, sea hares,molluscs, echinoderms, bryozoans, prawns, shells, sea slugs, marine microorganisms, and phytoplankton's. Such aquatic living organisms have been basically screened for antibacterial, cardioactive, immunomodulator, anti-fungal, anti-inflammatory, anticancer, antimicrobial, neuroprotective, analgesic, toxins, and antimalarial properties. Example – Zoranol and Iso-Zoranol obtained from marine algae have been used as antimicrobial agents, Simularin obtained from corals has been used as anticancer agents, Cucumechinoside-F obtained from sea cucumber has been used as an antiprotozoal, Eptatretin obtained from sea fish is a potent cardiac stimulant, Laminine obtained from marine algae is a hypotensive agent, Ciguatoxin, Tetrodotoxin& Palytoxin are potent marine toxins with effect on nervous and cardiovascular systems, and Bio-Indol obtained from marine cyanobacterium is a good anti-inflammatory agent.

Examples of clinically approved marine drugs: -Cytarabine (used in leukaemia), Vidarabine (used in recurrent epithelial keratitis caused by HSV), Ziconotide (analgesic), and Trabectedin (used for the treatment of ovarian cancer).

f) **Plant tissue culture**: It is an artificial method of growing plants (in-vitro multiplication of plant cells) in laboratory conditions on defined solid or liquid medium under aseptic conditions through various biotechnological interventions. Those plants whose production of secondary metabolites is very less can undergo genetic manipulation and can be made to produce 2-3 times more secondary metabolites when such plants are grown in laboratory conditions. Also, through such genetic manipulation pest resistant and frost-resistant plants can be produced. Example – production of catharanthine from *Catharanthus roseus*, Diosgenin from *Dioscorea doryphore*, reserpine from *Rauwolfia* species, Ginsenosides from *Panax ginseng* are some good examples of drugs obtained through the tissue culture method.

g) **Animal source:** drugs obtained from the animal source could be either in the form of the whole animal, glandular products like thyroid gland, liver extracts, secretions/fluids of animals, etc. Such products undergo several stages of purification and processing before human consumption. For example -the pancreas of animals is a source for insulin. The sheep thyroid gland is a source for thyroxin, animal blood (horse) is used for the preparation of some vaccines, cod-liver oil from sharks and honey from bees.

h) **Mineral source:** Bothe metallic and non-metallic minerals have been extensively used in traditional medicine since ancient times. Siddha system of medicine extensively uses animal products and minerals of metallic origin in their formulation. Minerals are required in the body in trace quantities to maintain the normal physiology of the body, and their deficiency can lead to various diseases or can complicate pre-existing diseases. For example – iron is used in iron deficiency anaemia, iodine is used in antiseptics, gold salts are used as an anti-inflammatory in the treatment of rheumatoid arthritis.

i) **Microbial source:** microbes are an important source of drugs. Most of the microbes (bacteria) that are used for the production of drugs are obtained from the soil. Microbes continually keep producing certain antibiotics and other biochemicals inside them to gain an advantage over other competitors in the microbial world in the quest for survival. These antibiotics or chemicals are extracted and used for drug development, particularly antibiotics. Microbes can be effectively used to produce antibiotics, vaccines and various therapeutically important enzymes and proteins which can be used as anti-tumour and immunosuppressants. Currently, genetically engineered microorganisms are used for the production of certain targeted biochemicals, which can be potential drug sources. Example- penicillin produced by *Penicillium chrysogenum*, streptomycin from *Streptomyces griseus*. Aminoglycosides such as gentamicin and tobramycin are obtained from streptomyces and micromonosporas.

32. Explain the process of selection of herbal materials for manufacturing herbal preparations.

In the case of organized farming, only those species which are authorized in pharmacopoeia or other government documents should only be used for cultivation. In the case of wild cultivation, genuine herbal materials free from adulteration needs to be selected. The herbal materials are selected at an appropriate vegetative stage when they are fully grown and contain the maximum amount of phytoconstituents. Since the quality of herbal preparations depends on the amount of phytoconstituents present in the finished product, henceforth, it becomes very important that the starting material (herbal materials) must be selected at an appropriate vegetative stage when it contains the maximum phytoconstituents. At the same time, selection of herbal materials should also be made at an appropriate season which favors maximum production of phytoconstituents. Examples,

- Leaves: are collected during the flowering period when the photosynthetic activity is at the maximum. The collection should be made duringdry season because the presence of moisture can cause the degradation of phytoconstituents.

- Flowers: are collected before their full blooming and just before the pollination. It should be collected in dry season because moisture on the petals may cause discolouration during drying.

- Barks: are collected in spring or during early summer when the cambium is active and easily separable. Some barks like those of wild cherry bark are collected in autumn.

- Roots and rhizomes: are collected when they are fully stored with food reserves and before the stoppage of the vegetative process.

33. List out the WHO recommended good processing practices used in making different herbal preparations.

a) The quality of the raw material should be in accordance with that mentioned in herbal pharmacopeia or other official books of that particular country.

b) Authentication of the herbal raw material is very important. If organized cultivation was undertaken, authenticated seeds should have been used, and if wild collection is undertaken, taxonomical, microscopical, macroscopical, and chemical authentication should be carried out.

c) Proper documentation of the herbal raw material should be made as specified in the WHO recommended GMP for herbals.

d) Requisite primary processing steps must be carried out, followed by drying and size reduction.

e) Storage time of herbal raw material should be reduced, and processing must take place at the earliest to avoid any contamination or microbe triggered degradation of phytoconstituents.

f) All operational steps involved in the making of herbal preparations from processed herbal material should be hygienic and as per standard operating procedures.

34. Explain the type of documentation involved as per WHO guidelines during the processing of herbal materials into herbal preparations.

During the processing of herbal raw materials, the records regarding the following should be made,

a) Details of the herbal material used, including its botanical name and plant part used

b) Stage of vegetative development when harvesting was performed

c) Cultivation site details

d) Details of the supplier of raw material

e) Drying details (if performed)

f) Details of primary processing performed along with dates of such operations carried out, including the details of the manpower (in-charge) involved in the process

g) The gross weight of the herbal material before and after processing

h) Involvement of any special processing

i) Master formula for the making of the herbal preparation

j) Details of usage of any animal-derived products or any adjuvants, if used

k) In-process control records along with records of batch production data

l) Records of quality control parameters of the finished product

m) Storage conditions

n) Shelf-life.

35. Write a note on organic farming.

Organic farming can be defined as that system of agricultural practice and management that is committed to the preservation of biodiversity, the ecosystem as a whole, and the well-being of humans and animals. It is based on the following principles,

a) The principle of health: Organic farming is committed to the preservation and enhancement of the health of soil, plant, animal, human, and planet as single system. It means thata healthy ecosystem shall provide healthy soil for the production of the healthy crop, which shall uphold the well-being of this planet by keeping humans and animals healthy. The basic role of organic farming is to maintain a healthy ecosystem and to ensure that all organisms in that ecosystem, starting from microbes in the soil to humans, should get high-quality, nutritious food. As a result, organic farming avoids the use of chemical fertilizers, pesticides, insecticides which may be harmful to the ecosystem on the whole.

b) The principle of ecology: Organic agriculture should achieve ecological balance through the design of farming systems, establishment of habitats and maintenance of genetic and agricultural diversity. Those who produce, process, trade, or consume organic products should protect and benefit the common environment, including landscapes, climate, habitats, biodiversity, air and water.

c) The principle of fairness: Organic agriculture should build on relationships that ensure fairness with regard to the common environment and life opportunities by ensuring the supply of good food quality and reduction of poverty among farmers

d) The principle of care: Organic agriculture should be managed in an accountable and responsible manner by not involving genetic engineering products so that the health and well-being of current and future generations and the environment arebeingmaintained.

Some of the good practices under organic farming are,

a) Non-usage of any synthetic chemicals in the form of fertilizers,or pesticides

b) Avoidance of concept of genetic engineering

c) Recycle of waste

d) Crop rotation for soil regeneration

e) Use of biopesticide and biological methods for pest control

f) Ensure suitable ecosystem for soil microorganisms and animals

g) Protection and maintenance of biodiversity.

Advantages of organic farming,

a) Produces vegetables with improved nutritive value

b) Produces medicinal plants with better yield of nutraceuticals and other secondary metabolites

c) Pesticide and heavy metal contamination is kept under acceptable limits

d) Lesser chances of inducing cancer risk in the future because of non-usage of synthetic chemicals

e) Consumption of organic products provide a better healthy life

f) Beneficial for the ecosystem on the whole as soil fertility and microbial flora of the soil is retained and also improved.

36. Write a short note on Biopesticides.

Biopesticides are those agents which are used to manage agricultural pests by means of specific biological effects rather than as broader chemical pesticides. It is a type of pest controlling product that makes use of biological resources, namely, natural organismsor ingredients obtained from natural materials (such as animals, plants, bacteria,or certain minerals), which also includes their genes or metabolites, for controlling pests.

Classification,

a) Microbial pesticides and other entomopathogens: pesticides that contain microorganisms like bacteria, fungi, or viruses, which attack specific pest species, or entomopathogenic nematodes. Mostly targeted for insect pests, but certain microorganisms are used for the eradication of weed. Examples – The bacterium *Bacillus thuringiensis*is used against caterpillars, and the fungus *Beauveria bassiana* is usedagainst whiteflies, aphids and thrips.

b) Plant protectants obtained through genetic manipulation: these include pesticidesubstances that are produced in genetically modified plants or organisms.

c) Biochemicals: these are plant-based extracts containing phytoconstituents which has pesticide properties. This includes insect repellents, pheromones, and plant growth regulators. Examples - Azadirachtin (broad-spectrum insecticide), Capsaicin (broad-spectrum insecticide, nematicide and fungicide), Clove, rosemary and peppermint oil (broad-spectrum fungicide).

Advantages,

- less toxic to humans and the environment
- do not leave harmful residues
- pest-specific agents
- capable of replication in target host and persist in the environment resulting in long-term suppression of pest populations even without repeating the application
- the sustainable component in Integrated Pest Management.

Disadvantages,

- since they are pest-specific, hence, cannot control a large species of pest
- have reduced shelf life because they contain living organisms
- efficacy is often variable due to the influence of various biotic and abiotic factors
- well informed manpower is required for usage of such products
- thorough knowledge regarding the target pest is required so that optimization regarding application time, field rates, and application intervals can be done
- biopesticides often are developed by research institutions rather than by the traditional pesticide industry. Hence large-scale commercial availability of such products can be an issue
- it is challenging to design an appropriate formulation for efficient field application.

37. Explain the basic principle of Ayurveda.

Ayurveda means 'The Science of life'. It is made of combination of two Sanskrit words 'Ayur' which means life and "Veda" which means knowledge. The fundamental doctrine principle of Ayurveda is based on the belief that the universe is composed of five basic elements, namely, Prithvi (earth), Vayu (air), Jala (water), Aakash (space) and Teja (fire). These five elements are known as Panchabhutas, which exists in the human body in the form of "Doshas', namely, Vata, Pitta and Kapha, collectively known as Tridosha (humour), which regulate the basic physiological functions of the body. In addition to this, the principle of Ayurveda also states the existence of seven basic elements known as 'Sapta dhatus' which are represented by Rasa (tissue fluids), Rakta (blood), Mamsa (muscle), Meda (fat & connective tissue), Asthi (bone), Majja (marrow), Shukra (semen) andMala(such as faeces, urine and sweat).Vata dosha takes care of cellular transport, electrolyte balance andelimination ofwaste products. Pitta dosha maintains body temperature, regulates optic nerve coordination along with hunger and thirst. Kapha is believed to maintain lubrication between joints. Vata is responsible for catabolism, Pitta for metabolism and Kapha for anabolism of the body. To maintain a healthy state of living, an optimal balance of the Doshas and other Sapta dhatus are required. Any imbalance shall give rise to a diseased condition. Apart from Doshas and Dhatus, Tri-Malas (urine faeces, sweat) also plays a vital role in maintaining healthy living as their routine excretion is very important to eliminate the toxins generated inside the body. A holistic approach is adopted in Ayurveda for the diagnosis of the disease where the patient as a whole is examined and not only just the symptoms. Ayurveda uses the 'PanchaKarma' mode of therapy, which is based on rejuvenation, cleansing of the body and increasing its longevity. This mode of therapy is composed of five karmas, namely, Virechan (purgation using decoctions), Vaman (forced emesis), Basti (enemas made from essential oil), Rakta moksha (removing toxins from the blood) and Nasya (administering drugs in suitable forms through nasal route). Pancha Karma consists of three steps namely, Poorvakarma (preparing the patient and medications to be used for treatment), Pradhan karma (the stage where the drug is actually administered) and Paschata karma (indicates post-treatment procedures).

38. Explain the basic principle of Siddha.

The word Siddha is derived from the 'Siddhi', which means achieving excellence, and this excellence in medicine was achieved by a group of eighteen saints known as 'Siddhars' who later spread the knowledge. Siddha is more prevalent in the Tamilian culture. The philosophy of Siddha is also similar to Ayurveda and follows the concept of Panchamahabhutas and Doshas. Matter and energy, which are also known as Siva and Sakthi, are believed to be the two most powerful components of the universe according to Siddha philosophy and plays a vital role in maintaining body's healthy condition. Apart from the balance of Doshas, according to the Siddha system, the well-being of the body is also regulated by 96 other factors, namely pulse, perception, speech etc. Diagnosis in the siddha system is carried out through 'Ashtasthana Pareeksha' which indicates the examination of eight sites of the body, namely pulse, eyes, voice, colour, tongue etc.Siddha system predominantly uses various metals (gold, silver, copper) and mineral-based preparations. Usage of herbs is less when compared to Ayurveda.

39. Explain the basic principle of Unani.

Unani system of medicine originated in Greece by Hippocrates and later on further developed by Galen and Aristotle. This system was introduced in India by Arabs and incorporated into the Indian mainstream of medicine by the Mughal emperors. Unani philosophy is based on four conditions of living represented as hot, sodden, frosty, and dry. It is also based on four senses of humour (namely- blood, yellow bile, dark bile, and mucus) as proposed by Hippocrates, whose balance is essential for body's healthy condition. Hippocrates also stated that balance among basic elements, humour and temperament are the minimum requirements for a healthy soul. The proper balance of these senses of humour is maintained by an intrinsic power of the body known as *Quwut-e-Modabira*. Weakening of this power will lead to an imbalance among the humor leading to the diseased condition. *Asbabe-Sita-Zarooriya* indicates six essential features required for the prevention of diseases, namely, air, food, drinks, body response, sleep, excretion and retention. Treatment protocol under Unani comprises of three basic strategies,

- Ilajbit-ghiza – diet therapy
- Ilajbit-tadbeer – regimental therapy
- Ilajbit-dawa – pharmacotherapy

40. Explain the basic principle of Homeopathy.

The word homeopathy has been derived from two Greek words, 'homeos' which means similar and 'pathos'which means suffering. Even though the concept originated in Greece by Hippocrates, modern-day homeopathy was developed by a German Physician Dr. Samuel Hahnemann. The principle of homeopathy is based on the similarity in terms of body's response to the drug and the disease. It uses medicines that produces similar symptoms to that of the disease, resulting in initial aggravation of the disease and then finally treating it. Two basic methodologies are involved,

a)   *Like cures Like*: if a drug (tincture) administered to a healthy person produces certain symptoms in the human body, then the same drug would be used for the treatment of those diseases which produced similar symptoms to that of the drug when given to a healthy person. Symptoms produced by the drugs in a healthy person = symptoms produced by a particular disease. In such a situation, both can neutralize the effects of each other. For example – extract of cinchona bark produces malaria-like symptoms when given to a healthy individual. Hence it was decided that such extract could be useful for the treatment of malaria.

b)   *Infinite dilution*: the therapeutic activity is enhanced upon successive dilutions, even if the dilution goes beyond the Avogadro's number.

41. Write a note on Arishta and Asava.

Asava-arishta is hydro-alcoholic ayurvedic formulation products generated through the traditional fermentation process. They are basically prepared by subjecting herbal juices or herbal decoctions to fermentation with the addition of sugar or jaggery. This particular dosage form results in neutralizing the toxic effects of various phytoconstituents or converting them into a more potent form apart from offering a better degree of bio-absorption. Moreover, the alcohol content also serves as an extraction solvent for dissolving out the phytoconstituents from the starting material and also act as a preservative. The process of making Asavas and Arishtas is known as 'Sandhana kalpana' in Ayurveda. General methods used in the extraction of medicinal plants in asava and arishta are infusion and decoction. Decoctions are the starting material for the preparation of Arishta, and fresh herbal juices are the starting material for Asavas. Flavouring agents may be added to alter the taste of the finished product. The medicinal plants used for such preparationare cleaned and pulverized. For Asavas, the juice is collected from a fresh plant using mechanical pressure, and if the dried crude drug is used, an infusion is prepared. For Arishta, a decoction is produced. Old jaggery or honey is then added and dissolved,which provides a medium for fermentation. Earthen pots whose internal surface is smeared with 'ghee' are used as fermentation containers. 'Ghee' blocks the natural perforation present in the earthen pot so that the inner contents are not exposed to outside air, which otherwise could affect the fermentation process. The reaction mixture (juices/infusion for Asavas or decoctions for Arishtas + honey or jaggery + flavouring agent + additional powdered drugs) is poured into the earthen pots upto three-fourth capacity so that during fermentation, increase in volume due to frothing and other gasses can be accommodated in the earthen pot. Yeasts are required as inoculum for initiating the fermentation. Hence, dhataki flowers (*Woodfordia fruticosa*) or mahua flowers are added.

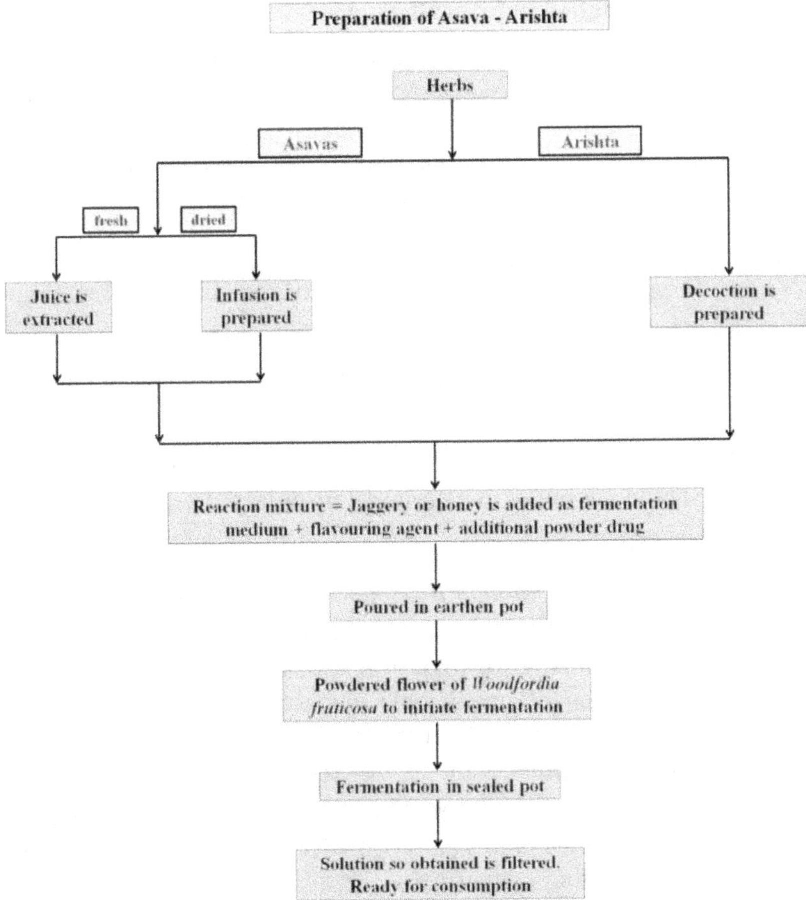

Finally, the vessel is sealed with clay smeared cloth. The vessel is to be kept in the dark place without much air circulation. It can be kept in a grain store or buried in a pit. The time to complete the fermentation depends on the season, summer season requires lesser time (6-7 days) and winter season requires maximum time (10-14 days). The fermentation vessel is generally left undisturbed for a month before opening and then filtered to separate the sediment. The filtrate serves as the finished product. Example – Ashokarishta (used in painful menstruation, relieves inflammation, and increases appetite) and Kanakasava(used in asthma and blood disorders).

42. Write a detailed note on Bhasmas.

Bhasmas are ayurvedic preparation obtained by the process of calcination (heating metals at high temperatures for conversion into their respective oxides) of metals (gold, silver, copper etc.) or minerals (calcium, magnesium, aluminium, zinc etc.) or animal products treated with herbal extracts.

Characteristics of Bhasma,

- A typical specified colour occurs for each bhasma preparation
- Should be lusterless (should not glow or appear shiny)
- Bhasma should be in powder form, light enough to float on still water surface
- Should not cause irritation to the mucous membrane
- Should not revert to its original metallic form
- It should be tasteless.

Method of preparation of Bhasma: it involves two steps, namely,

a) *Shodhana* (Purification): the basic objective of shodhana is the elimination of toxic properties of metals and minerals, conversion of undesirable characteristics of the drug and improving the overall therapeutic action. There are two types of shodhana,

- Saamanya shodhana: thin sheets of metals are heated and converted into coarse powder and repeatedly quenched into oil or cow urine

- Vishesha shodhana: involves certain special treatments like wet grinding of coarsely powdered metals with a specific liquid preparation – the process is known as *Bhaavana* and dipping of red-hot metal into liquids like oil – a process known as *Nirvaapana*.

b) *Marana*: the powdered metals obtained after purification is triturated with a specific extract. The contents are transferred to an earthen pot and sealed with clay smeared cloth. The vessel is then placed in a pit which is dug in the ground and surrounded with cow dung cakes which are then ignited to complete the burning (incineration) process. The whole process may be repeated several times. Finally, the bhasma so obtained is powdered and is ready for use. The above method is known as the *Putapaka method*. Bhasma may also be prepared by the *Kupipakwa method*, which involves an amalgamation of the purified metal with mercury followed by trituration with purified Sulphur. This preparation is known as *Kajjali*. Subsequently, the preparation is then subjected to wet grinding with a specified extract/liquid, dried and packed in a glass bottle, sealed and subjected to sand bath for homogenous heating. Finally, the bottle is broken, and bhasma is collected from the bottom and powdered.

Example – Swarna bhasma (analgesic activity, antioxidant), Loha bhasma (used in the treatment of jaundice and anemia) and Tamra bhasma (antioxidant in nature).

43. Write a brief note on *avaleha.*

Avaleha is an ayurvedic preparation obtained by continuous heating of an aqueous extract of a crude drug along with other medicaments and additives.

Basic ingredients of Avaleha = aqueous extract (Kashaya) of a crude drug + substrate (sugar/jaggery) + powdered drug + lipid medium (ghee/oil) + additives (honey).

According to the consistency of the final product, several synonyms are given, such as *Avaleha, Leha, Lehya, Avalehya, Rasakriya* etc.

Method of preparation: the aqueous extract of the crude drug is prepared, and sweetening agents like jaggery is mixed and heated over a mild fire in a stainless-steel vessel. The contents are cooled and filtered and heated again to a further thicker consistency. At this stage, ghee or oil is added. At this point, the preparation is known as *Paka lakshana*. Fine powder of other crude drugs is added to the mixture while hot and stirred to obtain a homogenous mixture and allowed to cool. Honey is added at the end, and the product is finally packed in air tight containers.

Example – Chyavanaprasa, Kushmanda Avaleha.

Ten marks category questions

44. **What do you mean by processing of herbal raw material? Explain in detail the different processing stages of herbal raw material.**

Processing of herbal raw materials indicates the application of some unique processes through which crude drugs collected from the field in raw form are converted into a suitable state so that they can be further used for,

- Storage for longer duration and transportation to distant places
- Making of herbal preparations followed by making of different herbal formulations or dosage forms
- Different industrial processing in accordance with GMP required for preparing herbal finished products
- Neutralizing the toxicity or enhancing the therapeutic activity of the drug
- Reduction of microbial contamination through the removal of moisture
- Convenience in packaging.

Thus, herbal processing means all those processes involved in the making of processed herbal materials to finished herbal products with the goal to assure quality at every stage. Processing involved in different stages starting from herbal raw materials to finished product (herbal medicine) is presented below,

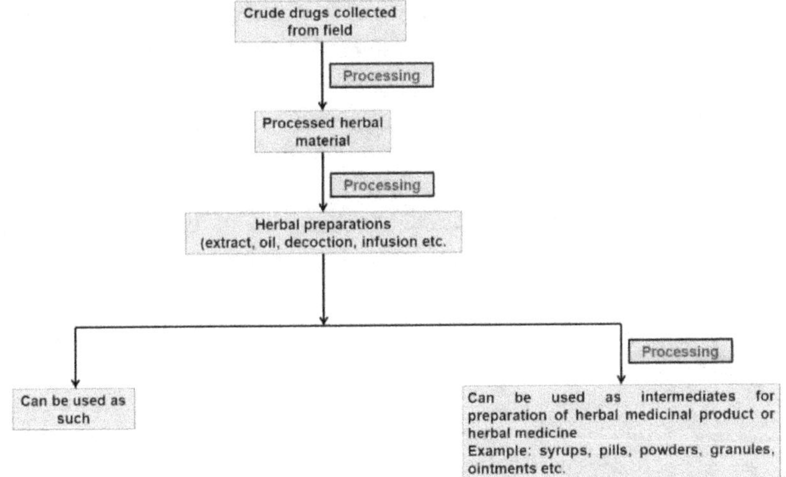

Processing of herbs at different stages,

Processing of raw materials (crude drugs) into herbal materials: this indicates the conversion of the raw form of the crude drug as obtained from nature into a form suitable for therapeutic application or further processing into herbal preparations. Various processing steps involved in this stage are,

Primary processing:

a) Harvesting: good harvesting practices should be adopted. Harvesting of plants should be done at the appropriate vegetative stage when the plant contains maximum phytoconstituents. Trained manpower and specific instruments should be used for harvesting to avoid any damage to the plant material during the process of harvesting.

b) Garbling: this is the first step after harvesting, where the plant material is cleaned, and all unwanted things like dirt, sand, soil, unwanted non-medicinal parts are removed and sorted. Sorting can be done using mechanical means (machines) or by hand through trained manpower.

c) Washing: washing with water (running tap water or chlorinated water) is recommended for cleaning additional dirt and soil adhering to the surface of the raw material. Herbal raw materials should not be soaked in water for a long period of time for the purpose of cleaning.

d) Blanching: herbal raw material dipped in boiling water for a short time period to facilitate removal of the seed coat of almonds, gelatinizing starch content etc. Such process improves the storage life of the raw material, reduces chances of mould or insect contamination and also deactivates certain enzymes whose activation otherwise could have degraded certain phytoconstituents.

e) Drying: this step is an essential component of the processing of herbal raw material. Mostly herbal raw materials are subjected to drying unless instructed to use fresh , particularly in case of extraction of essential oil, juices, resins and other exudates. Advantages of drying are,

- Removes moisture content, and thus microbial growth can be avoided

- Prevents tissue deterioration

- Prevents phytochemical alteration likely to be caused by activation of enzymes triggered by the presence of moisture

- Helps in size reduction so that the raw material can be subjected to further extraction process.

Major aspects of drying are,

- Temperature control
- Humidity
- Air flow
- Cleanliness of air
- Tissue structure and chemical constituents present and their sensitization towards drying
- The appearance of the final form post drying.

Based on the above-mentioned aspects, drying type is selected, which are as follows,

- *Sun-drying*: herbal raw materials should be spread out and subjected to natural sun-drying in the open air.

Necessary precautions must be taken to protect the raw material from pollution, dust, rain and other possible sourcesof contamination. The material should be turned upside down frequently to achieve uniform drying. Volatile oil-bearing plants are not subjected to direct sun-drying in the open air. Discolouration of the herbal raw material is very much possible.

- *Shade-drying*: herbal raw material spread in the thin layer can be subjected to shade drying with or without artificial airflow. Such drying process is slow but prevents discolouration or degradation of phytoconstituents.

- *Drying by means of artificial heat*: the temperature and humidity may be controlled depending upon the physical and chemical nature of the raw material. Temperature preferably may be kept below 50°C. Drying by artificial means can be conducted by Tray drying- drugs (roots and rhizomes) are spread across a tray, and hot air is circulated throughout the closed system, Vacuum drying- expensive method, used for drugs which are sensitive to temperature and humidity as well, Spray drying- liquid extract/exudate is introduced in fine mist form in a heating tower supplied with hot air. Moisture evaporates in a flush and converts the liquid feed into powder. E.g., preparation of powder for capsules and tablets.

  - *Microwave drying:* crude drugs can be dried by exposure to the microwave while moving in a closed system through a conveyer belt. The moisture absorbs the microwave, gets heated and evaporates.

  - *Infrared radiation drier:* crude drugs are subjected to infrared radiation while passing through a closed system, resulting in evaporation of the moisture present in the crude drug.

e) Storage: processed herbal raw materials should be stored in closed, dry and well-ventilated rooms duly protected from light and with appropriate humidity conditions to avoid any microbial growth. Contamination from other sources should also be avoided. The storage area should have sufficient capacity for accommodating all types of materials with a quarantine facility for those materials which require the same. Separate receiving and dispatch areas should be maintained.

Secondary processing:

f) Size reduction: herbal raw material is subjected to size reduction using machineslike a ball mill. Size reduction offers ease of manufacturing, improves extraction yield and ease in packaging and transportation.

g) Ageing: refers to storing the herbal raw material for a certain time period immediately after collection from the field. Example- cascara should be aged for one year prior to using in herbal preparations, which is necessary for removing the strong irritation effects that may cause vomiting.

h) Boiling or steaming: herbal raw material may be subjected to boiling water or steam. Prior treatment with wine or vinegar may be carried out before exposure to steam. This is necessary to denature certain enzymes or to thermally degrade certain chemical constituents. Example- boiling rhizomes of *Acorus calamus* in cow urine can enhance its anti-convulsant activity

i) Stir-frying: raw materials are put in a frying pan and continuously stirred for a certain period. Wine, vinegar, honey may be added during the stirring process. Stirring may continue until the external colour changes. Example- liquorice roots and rhizomes are often stirred with honey, fresh ginger is often stir-fried with sand.

j) Fumigation: fumigation by Sulphurdioxide has been often employed for the purpose of preserving the colour, preventing the growth of insects and also applied to herbal raw materials with bright colours to prevent browning.

Special processing

k) They are mainly done to reduce the toxic effects of certain phytoconstituents. Sometimes also carried out to enhance the therapeutic properties of a drug. For example- aconite and nux-vomica are generally boiled in water/steam to reduce their toxic effects. Fresh ginseng is converted to red ginseng, which has a better pharmacological activity by a series of steaming process.

Processing for conversion of processed herbal materials into herbal preparations:

Processed herbal materials may be used as herbal medicine as such or may be further processed to prepare different herbal preparations, which can further be used alone or in combination with processed herbal materials for making finished herbal medicinal products. All procedures adopted should be in accordance with WHO recommended GMP guidelines for herbals. For the making of herbal preparations, different extraction methods using different solvents and extraction conditions are employed to get the optimum yield. The most common herbal preparation is a herbal extract.

Herbal extracts: extracts are of four basic types,

   (i)   Liquid extract: it is a liquid preparation of herbal materials commonly using water or alcohol as the solvent. Some examples of the liquid extract are,

       Fluidextract - is an alcoholic liquid extract produced by percolation of herbal material,

       Decoction - Decoction is a water-based herbal preparation made by boiling herbal materials with water,

       Infusion- is a dilute solution made by subjecting the herbal materials in boiling water for a short time only,

       Tincture - it is an alcoholic or hydro-alcoholic extract.

   (ii)   Soft extract: it is a semi-solid preparation prepared by partial evaporation of the solvent from the main extract.

   (iii)   Oleoresin: type of semi-solid product consisting of resin mixed in a solution of essential oil.

(iv) Dry extract: solid extract in powder form obtained by complete evaporation of the extracting solvent using techniques like spray drying.

Processing for conversion of herbal preparations into finished herbal products or herbal dosage forms: Herbal preparations obtained after subjecting the processed herbal materials (botanical material) to processes like extraction can then be used as intermediates for the preparation of finished herbal products or herbal dosage forms. Such dosage forms or finished medicinal products, namely, syrups, ointments, tablets, capsules, creams etc., must be prepared under strict WHO recommended GMP conditions.

45. Explain in detail the methods used for the identification and authentication of herbal materials.

Identification of herbal raw materials indicates correct botanical and taxonomic identification of the plant species free from any possible adulterants. It is highly possible that during wild collection, a wrong plant species or a similar-looking plant may be collected by mistake, which will then badly affect the subsequent steps to follow in the preparation of the final finished herbal product. Identification can be made by a taxonomist by studying the botanical and reproductive features of the plant. Microscopic and phytochemical evaluations can also be done to identify the plant species. Authentication refers to a quality assurance process that validates the identification process carried out for choosing the correct herbal raw material and ensures the quality, safety and efficacy of the herbal material and finished product produced thereafter using the herbal raw material. Official pharmacopoeia of every country provides distinctive quality control procedures for performing identification cum authentication of herbal materials by comparison to standards mentioned in such official books. Such parameters are described below,

a) *Organoleptic evaluation (morphological evaluation):* refers to colour, odour, taste, arrangement of calcium oxalate crystals, aleurone grains, types of fibres, vessel thickenings, which, reveal vital information regarding the identification and authentication of herbal materials (Example – cinchona contains lignified bast fibres, nuxvomica contains lignified trichomes etc.). On the other hand, quantitative microscopy of drugs mainly includes stomatal index, vein-islet number, vein termination number and palisade ratio, which can be compared with reference value mentioned in official books, helps in differentiating closely similar-looking species, thus helps in avoiding possible adulteration. The above-mentioned terms are known as leaf constants, and their value is constant for a particular leaf species irrespective of the age and size of the leaf. Very useful in quality control of powdered drugs.

b) Foreign organic matter: any other plant parts or any other material other than those specified which does not constitute the desired herbal raw material (crude drug) are considered as foreign matter. Any matter of plant or animal, or mineral origin which is undesirable, constitutes the foreign matter. The collected crude drug should be free from soil, dust, earthy material or any type of animal or insect contamination, including animal excreta.

c) *Ash value*: upon incineration (not exceeding 600°C) of crude drugs, they leave inorganic ash which is an indication of the care taken during the processing of crude drugs, especially for underground drugs. There are three different ash values namely,

- Total ash: indicates the total ash obtained after incineration of the crude drug. It includes 'Physiological ash'which is derived from the burning of plant tissue, and, non-physiological ash'which is obtained by the burning of the extraneous undesirable material adhering to the crude drug surface like soil, sand and earthy material. Percent ash to be calculated with reference to the air-dried drug.

- Acid-insoluble ash: it is defined as the residue obtained after igniting the insoluble content resulting from boiling the total ash in dilute HCl. The high value of acid-insoluble ash indicates the excess presence of sand.

- Water-soluble ash: it is defined as the difference in weight between the total ash and the residue obtained after treating the total ash with water.

d) Extractive values: it refers to the percent chemical constituents (extractable matter) extracted from the crude drug using a specific organic solvent. It provides information regarding the extent of polar, non-polar and medium polarity constituents present in the crude drug. Since HPTLC/HPLC/GC instrumentation provides exact quantification of the active constituents present in the crude drug, henceforth, extractive values are of lesser significance in modern time. But still, it is an inexpensive and quick indicator of the exhaustive and adulterated drug. Alcohol and water extractive value must be determined.

e) Determination of moisture content: this parameter indicates the moisture content of the crude drug. The moisture content of a crude drug must be within specified limits because excess moisture content may encourage microbial growth leading to the deterioration of active constituents of crude drugs.The test specimen is to be dried at 105° C for 3 hours and then weighed. Drying and weighing are to be continued at half an hour intervals until the difference between two successive weighings corresponds to not more than 0.25%.

f) Chromatographic fingerprinting: this is a sure shot method for identification and authentication of herbal materials (crude drugs). Chromatographic fingerprint refers to a fixed chromatographic pattern indicating the presence of various active phytoconstituents or classes of phytoconstituents present in that extract obtained through the use of analytical instruments, namely, HPTLC, HPLC, GC-FID. A chromatographic pattern for an extract is usually fixed, and a standard chromatographic pattern for most of the commercial crude drugs are available in standard books. The similarity of the chromatographic pattern for the sample is matched with that of the standard for assessing its quality. A chromatographic fingerprint obtained from HPTLC is represented in the form of bands viewed under UV or fluorescent light, where each band represents a particular phytoconstituent. The intensity of the bands is matched. In the case of fingerprinting obtained through HPLC or GC, an array of peaks is obtained. A standard set of peaks obtained from a reference sample is considered as a standard chromatogram documented in official books. The set of peaks obtained from the test sample is matched with the chromatogram mentioned in official books. However, this test is a qualitative test where information regarding the quantity of phytoconstituents present in the extract is not reflected. Nevertheless, matching the chromatographic pattern provides conclusive evidence regarding the identity and authentication of the herbal raw material.

g) Pesticide residue: Pesticides are defined as any substance which is intended for preventing, destroying, attracting, repelling, or controlling any pest, including unwanted species of plants or animals during production, storage, transport, distribution and processing. Medicinal plants can easily accumulate pesticides through groundwater, soil and direct foliar application. World Health Organization has set maximum residuelimits of pesticides in medicinal plants. Different types of pesticides are dichlorodiphenyltricholoroethane (DDT), benzene hexachloride (BHC), toxaphene, aldrin, carbaryl etc. Extraction and sample enrichment of pesticide from herbal raw materials can be performed using solid-phase extraction, QuEChERS method etc. Quantification can be done by using GC, MS, GC-MS or immunochemical methods. Limit for DDT – 1 mg/Kg, aldrin – 0.05 mg/Kg.

h) Radioactive contamination: A certain amount of exposure to ionizing radiation is unavoidable because many sourcesof radionuclides occur naturally in the ground and the atmosphere. Examples of such radionuclides include long-lived and short-lived fission products, actinides and activation products. In general, the nature and the intensity of these radionuclides may differ markedly and depends on factors such as the source, which could be a reactor, reprocessing plant, fuel fabrication plant, isotope production unit or other. Instruments used for such detection are Geiger Mueller (GM) Detectors, Alpha Radiation Survey Meter, Dose Rate Meter etc.

i) Mycotoxin determination: Mycotoxins are secondary metabolic products that are non-volatile, having low molecular weight and are usually secreted onto or into the medicinal plant material. They help in eliminating other microorganisms competing in the same environment and, secondly, help parasitic fungi to invade host tissues. Mycotoxins produced by species of fungi including *Aspergillus, Fusarium and Penicillium* are the most commonly reported. Mycotoxins are of four major types, namely, aflatoxins, ochratoxins, fumonisins and trichothecenes, all of which have toxic effects. Permissible limit for B1 aflatoxin < 2ppb and for B1+B2+G1+G2 aflatoxin is < 5ppb.

j) Heavy metal contamination determination: due to environmental pollution and industrialization,it is very likely that medicinal plants may get contaminated with heavy metals like arsenic, cadmium, lead and mercury. For authentication of herbal raw materials, prescribed limits in parts per million should be satisfied. Permissible limits for lead are 10 ppm, arsenic – 3 ppm, cadmium – 0.3 ppm and mercury – 1 ppm. Atomic absorption spectrophotometry and the Indictive Coupled Plasma method can be used for determination of heavy metals.

k) Microbial contaminants: Herbs and herbal materials generally possess a large number of bacteria and molds which originates from soil or are derived from manure. Poor practices of harvesting, production, transportation and storage may cause additional contamination and microbial growth. Such microbial growth is mainly due to uncontrolled moisture levels in herbal materials. The presence of *Escherichia coli, Salmonella* and molds in herbal materials may possibly indicate poor production and harvesting practices. Microbial contamination may occur during harvest by personnel who are themselves infected with pathogenic bacteria, post-harvest processing and the manufacturing process. Total aerobic count, total fungal count and total Enterobacteriaceae count must be carried out using validated pharmacopoeia methods. The total count of *E. coli, Staphylococcus aureus, P. aeruginosa, Shigella* species and *Salmonella typhimurium* must also be determined.

46. What do you mean by Good Agricultural Practices (GAP)? Explain the WHO guidelines related to GAP in the cultivation of medicinal plants.

A GAP is defined as a well strategized cultivation protocol designed to ensure optimal yield in terms of both quality and quantity of any crop intended for health purposes.

Objectives of GAP:

- To improve the quality, safety and efficacy of finished herbal products by ensuring the quality of medicinal plant materials which are used as raw materials in the production of herbal medicine

- Lay down standard operating guidelines for good collection practices of medicinal plants

- To promote sustainable cultivation and collection of medicinal plants

- To support the conservation of medicinal plants and the environment at large

GAP Related to soil & climatic conditions:

a) Based on metrological data, the best suitable site for cultivation must be selected to ensure an optimal cultivation environment for plant growth both in terms of quality and quantity.

b) Sites having salinity, acidity factors in the soil, issues related to industrial waste disposal, graveyards, crematoria in close vicinity of cultivation site should be avoided.

c) The site should be asclose as possible to the source of irrigation.

d) Soil should be fertile and well-drained with good water holding capacity for providing the proper environment for plant growth. Latest reports on soil nutrients and other physico-chemical properties of the soil must be obtained to decide regarding the fertility status of the soil and take necessary corrective measures to improve fertility.

e) The quality of water used for irrigation, should be tested for the presence of heavy metals, pesticides and their levels should be within acceptable limits.

f) Availability of shades across the field, if required, may be ascertained.

g) Average rainfall, temperature, day & night temperature differences should be considered before cultivation.

GAP Related to seed and propagation material:

a) Correct identification of the seed/planting material is mandatory

b) Marker-based analytical projection for the end product is mandatory

c) Seeds to be used for cultivation must be physically free from pests and other diseases.

d) Seeds used should be fresh and must have originated from recent harvests

e) Applicable seed pretreatment procedures, if any, should be carried out well in advance before the planting season

f) If seedlings are required, they should be produced under nursery conditions as per standard agronomic practices well before the actual field transplantation.

GAP in crop management for cultivation:

a) Field preparation: includes providing proper physical conditions of the soil, better rhizospheric environment so that a nutritious environment for the plant can be created, which shall include the advantages of beneficial microorganisms also, good soil porosity & texture and eradication of weeds.

b) Sowing and transplantation:

- Seedlings per unit area of land shall be as per norms
- Proper spacing in terms of row-to-row and plant-to-plant
- Seedlings at the proper growth stage shall be transplanted to the field.

c) Manures and fertilisers:

- Organic manure shall be preferred
- Use of compost, vermicompost, green leafy manure is desirable
- Use of nitrogen-fixing bacteria
- Specialized nutritional care for distinct root production or enhancement of leafy bio-mass is desirable
- Any agrochemicals used to promote the growth of plants should be kept to a minimum level
- Only approved pesticides and herbicides shall be applied
- All applications of agrochemicals must be documented.

GAP in irrigation:

a) Total water requirements of the crop should be estimated, and accordingly, the irrigation cycles should be planned.

b) Water harvesting and water conservation methods should be followed.

GAP in harvesting:

a) Harvesting should take place in optimal season

b) Time of harvest depends on the plant part used

c) The best time of harvest should be determined according to the quality and quantity of biologically active constituents and not on the vegetative yield

d) During harvest, care should be taken to ensure that no foreign matter is mixed with the harvested medicinal plant materials

e) Harvesting shall be avoided during heavy dew, rain and high humidity conditions

f) Harvesting instruments and containers must be clean and free from any contamination

g) Any mechanical damage to harvested plant material during the filling of sacks or bags caused due to overfilling must be avoided.

GAP for personnel:

a) Personnel involved in cultivation must have thorough knowledge about the medicinal plant being cultivated.

b) All personnel involved in harvesting must be trained and properly equipped with all appropriate machinery and personnel protective gear required for harvesting.

c) All personnel involved in harvesting must maintain personnel hygiene.

47. Explain in detail the different methods of pest management.

The different methods of pest management are,

a) *Physical methods.* Such methods do not use any chemicals and include manual removal of pests or installing barriers between the crop and the pests. Generally, applicable for larger pests like rodents. Physical detection of the pests is made, and then various methods are adopted for their eradication like, manual collection of eggs and larvae of insects, trapping of rodents, cutting off branches which gather grasshoppers and other insects etc.

b) *Chemical methods*: includes the usage of various insecticides, pesticides and other chemicals mixed with water and sprayed on the leaves. This method is useful for the killing of those pests which generally cannot be seen easily and are difficult to remove by mechanical or physical methods. Pesticides kill pest through various mechanisms such as enzyme inhibition, disruption of signalling system, disruption of cellular components and membrane structures and altering the internal pH & osmotic balance. Such chemicals tend to accumulate in the crop and get potentially transferred to humans through the food chain, causing various neurological and hormonal disorders. Continuous use of the same pesticides can also lead to pesticide-resistant pests.

c) *Biological methods*: it involves the use of living organisms in the form of predators, pathogens or parasites, which shall provide a competitive environment for the pest and challenge its survival. Thus the abundance of pests in the field can be well regulated. There are three types of biological control (a) importation - the natural enemies of the pest are promoted through rearing or periodic release into the agricultural field, (b) augmentation – the natural enemy of the pest are bred and reared in large numbers and released into the infected crops to reduce the population of the pest, a process known as augmentation. Conservations refer to maintaining enough soil conditions for conserving the ecosystem of the natural enemies of the pest, (c) Importation - refers to the introduction of a pest's natural enemy to a new habitat where such natural enemies do not occur naturally. Example - release of parasitic wasps to control aphids.

d) *Cultural methods*: includes manipulating agricultural methods to control and avoid pest damage. In this case, pests are not directly killed, but due to adoption of simple agricultural or field practices at suitable times can result in a reduction of the pest population. Simple methods like crop rotation, deep ploughing, good preparation of soil, multiple cropping and intercropping with aromatic herbs are some simple techniques that makes the environment less favourable for pests and more favourable for natural enemies.

e) *Genetic methods*:   there are four strategies through which control over pests can be achieved

   • Sterile insect methods: a large number of sterile insects are released into the wild population as a method of pest control. Insects are made sterile by crosses between hybrid species or different genetic strains or by exposing the insects to ionization radiation to induce lethal mutations resulting in chromosomal damage and thus causing sterility. When such sterile 'insects' mate, the resulting eggs do not hatch because of the damage induced in the genetic material of the parents. Sufficient sterile insects must be released to achieve a significant decrease in the pest population over time. Once the healthy insects complete their life cycle, the future generation of pests shall not develop because of damage induced in their genetic material resulting in the non-hatching of their eggs.

   • Through various biotechnological interventions like gene editing, several genetically modified strains of pest species have been developed with lethality that operates only on females

- Transgenic plants express insecticidal toxins, which act against pests and prevents any pest mediated damage to the plant. Example – Bt toxins are expressed in Bt cotton against lepidoptera.

- Producing and release of transgenic male insects (carrying genes that are lethal on females) with severe lethal effects on females.

48. Explain the standardization parameters for arishtas and asavas.

The following standardization guidelines have been provided by AYUSH Ministry for standardization of arishtas and asavas,

a) Description: botanical description of the crude drug, including organoleptic and microscopic examination.

b) Colour: the final product should display the characteristics colour.

c) Odour: final product should display the characteristics odour.

d) pH: can be determined potentiometrically by using a glass electrode, a reference electrode and a pH meter.

e) Specific gravity: it is defined as the weight of a given volume of a liquid at 25°C compared with the weight of an equal volume of water at the same temperature. Weight is taken by pouring the liquid and water separately in a pycnometer.

f) Boiling point: the boiling range of a liquid is the range of temperature within which the whole or a specified portion of the liquid starts distilling at normal atmospheric pressure.

g) Refractive index: The refractive index is measured with reference to the wavelength of the D line of sodium (589.3 nm). Abbe's refractometer is used for the determination of refractive index.

h) Optical rotation: it is defined as the angle through which the plane of polarised light is rotated when polarised light obtained from sodium or mercury vapour lamp passes through one decimeter thick layer of a liquid or a solution of a substance at a temperature of 25°C. Substances are indicated as dextrorotatory or laevorotatory according to the clockwise or anticlockwise rotation. A polarimeter instrument is used for the determination of optical rotation.

i) Viscosity: indicates resistance to flow. Poise is the unit of dynamic viscosity.

j) Total solids: it is determined by taking 50 mL of asava and arishta in an evaporating dish, evaporated to dryness followed by drying at 105°C for 3 hours. The dish is to be weighed after cooling. The weight of the dried residue should be within prescribed limits as mentioned in specific official monograph.

k) Alcohol content: ethanol content is defined as the volume of ethanol contained in 100 volumes of the liquid, at 24.9°C – 25.1°C. Value is expressed as 'percent ethanol by volume'. It may also be expressed as gm of ethanol per 100 gm of liquid. Alcohol content can be determined by gas chromatography and the distillation method. In the case of gas chromatography, 5% v/v ethanol and 5% v/v 1-propanol are used as internal standards. From the distillation method, the specific gravity of the collected distillate is calculated and compared with the standard alcoholometric chart to find out the strength of the alcohol obtained from distillation.

l) Reducing sugar and non-reducing sugar.

m) TLC/HPTLC/GC-MS (anyone or all): comparison of the spots or bands in TLC/HPTLC with authenticated fingerprint under 254 nm or 366 nm can be done. Matching of R_f value with that of the standard mentioned in the monograph and intensity of spots/bands can serve as a semi-quantitative measurement for determining the chemical profile of the crude drug or finished formulation. GC-MS shall reveal peaks that can be identified using MS interface for determining the chemical profile of the herbal materials involved and the final finished product.

n) Test for methanol: can be determined using gas chromatography using column made of porous polymer beads and nitrogen as the carrier gas. Injection port temperature to be maintained at 170°C. Methanol 0.25% v/v and 1-propanol 0.25% v/v are used as internal standards.

o) Total acidity: sample is mixed with carbon dioxide-free water and titrated against standard sodium hydroxide solution using phenolphthalein as the indicator till persistence pink colour is observed. Water to be used as blank.

$$\text{Acidity as formic acid (\%) by weight} = \frac{0.23 \times V}{M}$$

V = corrected volume of 0.05N NaOH, M= weight in grams of sample taken

p) Test for heavy metals: the limits prescribed are, lead – 10 ppm, cadmium – 0.3 ppm, mercury – 1 ppm and arsenic – 3 ppm. Atomic absorption spectroscopy and Inductive coupled plasma detection may be used for the quantification of heavy metals.

q) Pesticide residue: presence of organochlorine pesticides, organophosphoras pesticides, and pyrethroids should be within prescribed limits as per ASU pharmacopoeia. A QuEChERS (Quick, Easy, Cheap, Effective, Rugged and Safe) based extraction method with GC-MS detection is one of the commonly used methods for the detection of pesticide residues.

r) Microbial contamination: limits prescribed in ASU pharmacopoeia are – the complete absence of *Staphylococcus aureus*, *Salmonella species*, *Pseudomonas aeruginosa*, *Escherichia coli*. Total microbial plate count (TPC) limits are 10^5/g (for herbal extracts) and 10^7/g (for topical applications). The total Yeast and Mould plate count limit is – 10^3/g.

s) Aflatoxins: they are poisonous and carcinogenic substances produced by certain fungi. The two most closely related species which produces most of the aflatoxins are *Aspergillus flavus* and *Aspergillus parasiticus*. Approximately there are 14 types of aflatoxins, out of which B_1, B_2, G_1 and G_2 are the most troublesome to human and animal health as they contaminate most of the crops and food materials. HPLC-MS and ELISA are mostly used for the detection of aflatoxins. Limits prescribed in ASU pharmacopoeia are $B_1 < $ 2ppb and B_1, B_2, G_1 and $G_2 < $ 5 ppb.

t) Shelf life: shelf life indicates the tenure for which the product is stable in terms of quality and efficacy under changing environments of temperature, humidity and light. It can be estimated by subjecting the finished herbal products of the same batch to standard storage conditions and accelerated storage conditions.

49. Explain the standardization parameters for ayurvedic churnas.

a) Description

b) Colour

c) Odour

d) Foreign matters: the sample (herbal material or herbal preparation) should be free from any visible signs indicating presence of mold, sliminess, stones, animal excreta, insects or any other undesirable matter. Take 100 g of the sample and spread it as a thin layer in a tray. Perform a careful examination under daylight. Suspected particles can be examined under 10x objective of a compound microscope.

e) Powder microscopy: powder sample can be used for performing standard detection tests associated with starch, lignified characters, determination of leaf constants, mucilage etc.

f) Loss on drying / Moisture content: it indicates the moisture content of the drug. 10 gm of the powder is taken in a tared petri dish and dried at 105°C in an oven for 5 hours. The sample is cooled for 30 min and weighed; the process is repeated until a constant weight not varying by more than 0.25% is obtained. Excessive moisture can lead to microbial growth, causing degradation of phytoconstituents. Henceforth, the determination of moisture content is an important quality control step.

g) Total ash and acid-insoluble ash: ash value indicates the presence of earthy material, dirt and sand along with the drug and must be within specified limits as prescribed in individual monographs. Higher ash value indicates possible adulteration of the drug with the above-said material, which is more frequent for underground plant parts like roots and rhizomes. Acid insoluble ash indicates the presence of sand or siliceous particles. Incinerate 2-3 g of the powder placed in a silica crucible at a temperature not exceeding 450°C until free from carbon. Calculate the weight of the total ash. For acid-insoluble ash, treat the total ash with 25 mL dilute HCl. Filter the mixture through ashless filter paper. Wash the residue on the filter paper with water until the filtrate is neutral. Dry the residue and ignite to a constant weight. Calculate the content of the acid-insoluble ash with reference to the air-dried drug.

h) pH

i) Water-soluble and alcohol soluble extractive: indicates the total extractable matter of the drug. Monographs specifieslimits for extractive values for different drugs. Five g of the powder is macerated with 100 mL chloroform water/alcohol in a closed flask for 24 hours with stirring for the first 6 hours. Twenty five mL of the filtrate is evaporated and dried at 105°C to a constant weight. The percent water-soluble extractive or alcohol-soluble extractive is calculated with reference to the air-dried drug.

j) Bulk density and tap density: The bulk density of a powder is the ratio of the mass of an untapped powder sample and its volume, including the contribution of the inter-particulate void volume. Hence, the bulk density depends onthe density of powder particles and the spatial arrangement of particles in the powder bed. The bulk density is expressed in g/ml and Kg/m^3 (1 g/ml = 1000 kg/m^3). The tapped density is an increased bulk density achieved after mechanically tapping a container containing the powder sample. The tapped density is obtained by mechanically tapping a graduated measuring cylinder containing the powder sample. After observing the initial powder volume or mass, the measuring cylinder is mechanically tapped, and volume or mass readings are taken.

k) HPTLC/HPLC with markers: fingerprint comparison should be done, and estimation of marker compounds should be carried out, and their levels must be above the minimum prescribed values mentioned in the individual monographs.

l) Test for heavy metals

m) Pesticide residue

n) Microbial contamination

o) Test for aflatoxins

p) Shelf life.

Brain Teasers (for competitive exams)

1. **How many Doshas are mentioned in Ayurveda?**

   Three, Vata, Pitta and Kapha

2. **Panchakarma mode of therapy is applicable for which system of medicine?**

    Ayurveda

3. **Practioners of Siddha are known as?**

    Siddhars

4. **In which state Siddha is more prevalent?**

    Tamilnadu

5. **Which country did Unani originate from?**

    Greece

6. **The importance of *Mijaz* for maintaining a healthy body is explained in which system of medicine?**

    Unani

7. **Practioners of Unani are known as?**

    Hakim

8. **Powdered drugs, when made in the shape of tablets, used as ayurvedic formulations are known as?**

    Vatika

9. **Powdered drugs, when made in the shape of pills used as ayurvedic formulation, are known as?**

    Gutika

10. **What is the starting material for asavas?**

    Juice extracted from fresh plant part or infusion prepared from dried crude drug

11. **What is the starting material for arishta?**

    Decoction prepared from dried crude drug

12. **The outcome obtained when herbal materials are subjected to various extraction methods is known as?**

    Herbal preparations (extract, decoctions, votalite oil etc.)

13. **Botanical Survey of India is located in which city?**

    Kolkata

14. **What is added to asavas and arishtas for initiating the fermentation process?**

    Fried flowers of *Woodfordia fruticose* (dhataki flowers)

15. **Which traditional system of medicine predominantly uses metals and minerals?**

Siddha

16. **What metals are frequently used in bhasmas?**

Gold, silver, copper and iron

17. **Name the microorganisms whose limits are prescribed in ASU pharmacopoeia?**

*Staphylococcus aureus, Salmonella species, Pseudomonas aeruginosa*and *Escherichia coli*

18. **Name the heavy metals whose limits are prescribed in ASU pharmacopoeia?**

Arsenic, cadmium, lead and mercury

19. **At what temperature loss on drying test is performed?**

105°C

20. **What type of ayurvedic preparation is Chyavanaprasa?**

Avaleha

21. **Which method of pest control makes use of ionizing radiation?**

Genetic method

22. **Which of the following leaf constants does not change with leaf size or age and is constants for a particular species?**

Stomatal index, Palisade ration, Vein-islet number and Vein-termination number

23. **Which ayurvedic formulation represents a form of nanomedicine?**

Bhasma

24. **'Law of Similar'or 'Like cures Like' is associated with which system of traditional medicine?**

Homeopathy

25. **Name the apparatus used for the determination of volatile matter?**

Clevenger apparatus

26. **Name the method used for the determination of alcohol content?**

Distillation and Gas chromatography

27. **Which carrier gas is used in gas chromatography for the determination of alcohol content?**

    Nitrogen

28. **The high value of acid-insoluble ash indicates?**

    Presence of excessive sand (silicious matter) as an adulterant in the crude drug

29. **Who is the founder father of Siddha?**

    Agasthya

30. **How many spores are present in each mg of lycopodium powder?**

    94000

31. **What is the formula of the stomata index?**

    S.I = S / E+S

32. **Aflatoxins are mostly produced by?**

    Fungus

Nutraceuticals, Herb-Drug and Herb-Food Interactions

Two marks category questions

1. **Name five Nutraceutical producing companies.**

   a) Sigma – Aldrich

   b) Novozymes

   c) Hester Bioscience

   d) Biosync Pharma

   e) Nivoxaa Biotech India Pvt. Ltd

2. **List out the health benefits of nutraceuticals.**

   a) It prevents chronic diseases and also helps in the management of existing lifestyle diseases

   b) Delays ageing

   c) Supports physiological and maintains the integrity of the body

   d) Enhances immunity

   e) Acts as anti-allergic

   f) Facilitates cell proliferation, antioxidant defence, gene expression, and safeguards mitochondrial integrity

   g) Effective in management of oxidative stress disorders.

3. **Define Dietary supplements.**

   Dietary supplements are those products (excluding tobacco) that include one or more of the following dietary ingredients: Vitamin, mineral, herb(s) or other botanicals, amino acid, and any other substance used to supplement the diet by increasing the total dietary intake. Nutraceuticals or functional foods are also included in dietary supplements. Example – Vitamins like B12,

C, E and D, minerals like calcium, various herbs like green tea and probiotics.

4. Who coined the term Nutraceutical?

The term nutraceutical was coined from "nutrition" and "pharmaceutical" in 1989 by Stephen DeFelice, founder and chairman of the *Foundation for Innovation in Medicine*

5. Name three types of nutrients and functional foods used in the management of diabetes.

Nutrients: Chromiun, magnesiun, vanadium

Functional foods: *Allium cepa* (Onion), *Eugenia jambolana* (Jamun), *Momordica charantia* (Bitter Gourd)

6. List out the mechanisms by which various nutraceuticals exhibits anticancer activity.

a)   Inactivation of NF-κB and other metastatic genes.

b)   Induction of apoptosis

c)   Change in cellmorphology andgrowth inhibition

d)   Alters the cell cycle

e)   It inhibits growth byinhibiting hedgehogsignalling pathways.

f)   Antioxidant activity

g)   Inhibits cell proliferation via caspase mediated cytotoxicity.

7. Name some phytochemical nutraceuticals, which are chemo-preventive and chemotherapeutic agents.

a)   Curcumin

b)   Quercetin

c)   Isoflavones of Soy protein

d)   Genistein

e)   Capsaicin

f)   Resveratrol

g)   Lycopene

8. Name four phytoconstituents used in the treatment of GI disorders.

a)   Curcumin

b)   Capsaicin

c)   Silymarin

d)   Quercetin

9.   **What do you mean by Functional food?**

Food provides basic nutrition and satisfies the body's metabolic needs. However, some groups of foods, in addition to their nutritional properties, also provide other additional health benefits. Such types of foods are called functional foods. Hence, functional food may be defined as any food that, apart from providing basic nutrition, also ensures good well-being for the person who consumes it. The ideal properties of functional foods are

- Theyshould be food and not a pharmaceutical formulation like a tablet or capsule derived from natural products.

- It should be consumed as a part of the daily diet.

- It has a particular function when eaten, serving to regulate a particular body process, such as enhancement of immunity, improving body's oxidative status, improving physical and mental health status, delays ageing etc.

10.   **Define probiotics, prebiotics and synbiotics.**

Probiotics are live microorganisms that, if administered in an adequate amount, provide a health benefit to the host. Probiotics may exert a beneficial effect on several pathogenetic pathways associated with irritable bowel syndrome, including the restoration of altered gut microbiota by increasing the number of beneficial bacteria's (like *Lactobacilli*) and reducing the number of pathogens because of competition. This combined effect leads to a decrease of inflammation caused due to the proliferation of pathogenic bacteria and restoration of normal colonic fermentation. Example - *Saccharomyces cerevisiae* strains are taken as probiotics in irritable bowel syndrome symptoms.

Prebiotics are defined as non-digestible, fermentable dietary components that exert beneficial effects on the host through the modulation of composition or activity of gut microbiota. For example - short-chain fructo-oligosaccharides improves digestive discomfort associated with patients having irritable bowel syndrome.

Synbiotics are dietary supplements that consists of a combination of prebiotics and probiotics. It increases the levels and activity of beneficial microbes in the gut. For example - a mixture of *Lactobacillus acidophilus, Lactobacillus helveticus and Bifidobacteria* in a medium enriched with phytoextracts is a synbiotic preparation that relieves pain and bloating in patients with irritable bowel syndrome.

11. **Name the class of phytoconstituents used for the treatment of constipation. Indicate its mechanism.**

Constipation is a common GI disorder which causes inadequate bowel movement or hardness of passing intestinal contents. Anthraquinone class of phytoconstituents are used widely for the treatment of constipation. The herbal drugs which contain anthraquinone derivates are Senna, Rhubarb, Cascara etc. Anthraquinone class of drugs exerts its effect by alteration of motility patterns and increase of colonic fluid volume leading to softening of stool and its easy passage.

12. **Name the enzymes present in honey.**
    a) diastase (amylase): converts starch or glycogen into smaller sugar units
    b) invertase (sucrase, α-glucosidase): converts sucrose into fructose and glucose
    c) glucose oxidase: converts glucose into hydrogen peroxide and gluconic acid
    d) catalase: converts peroxide to water and oxygen
    e) esterase: breaks ester bonds
    f) proteases: proteolytic enzymes
    g) β-glucosidase: converts β-glucans to oligosaccharides and glucose

13. **Name a marine nutraceutical source and mention its nutraceutical constituents.**

Marine source: blue-green algae found in seawater which consists of two most important species, namely, *Spirulina maxima* and *Spirulina platensis*, belonging to the family Oscillatoriacea.

- Carbohydrates: Mesoinositol phosphate

- Proteins: Contains all the essential amino acids
- Lipids: gamma-linolenic acid, linoleic acid and palmitic acid
- Vitamins and minerals: Vitamin B12, B1, B2, vitamin C, vitamin D and vitamin E. Rich in minerals like iron, calcium, chromium, copper
- Pigments: chlorophyll, phycocyanin and β-carotene
- Antioxidants: carotenoids such as astaxanthin
- Enzymes: rich in antioxidant enzyme superoxide dismutase enzyme.

14. What do you mean by herb-drug interaction and mention its consequences?

Co-administration of synthetic and herbal drugs leads to herb-drug interaction. Patients suffering from chronic illness and on a fixed medication with allopathic drugs often tend to take herbal drugs for small ailments or for managing the side effects caused by long term use of synthetic drugs. In such cases, herb-drug interaction is very common.

Consequences of herb-drug interactions:
- increased therapeutic or adverse effects
- decreased therapeutic or adverse effects
- any unique response that does not occur wheneither drug is used alone.

Consequences are both pharmacokinetic and pharmacodynamic in nature. An increase in bioavailability may lead to adverse toxic effects in patients, particularly in those drugs which have a narrow therapeutic window. Antagonistic effect shall cause a decrease in efficacy, resulting in failure of the therapy, which shall further worsen the diseased status of the patient. Example – interaction between warfarin (anticoagulant) and aspirin.

15. Write a note on the possible drug interactions of pepper.

Piperine is a major alkaloid present in *Piper nigrum*. Piperine may increase plasma concentrations of carbamazepine and diclofenac through inhibition of CYP3A4 enzyme (class of CYP enzymes). Administration of piperine modestly increases phenytoin plasma concentrations. Piperine inhibits P-glycoprotein, thus increasing fexofenadine bioavailability.

Five marks category questions

1. **Define nutraceuticals and give its detailed classification with examples.**

Nutraceutical is a substance that may be considered a food or part of food that provides medical or health benefits, including the prevention and treatment of diseases. Such products may include plant-based bioactives, dietary supplements, herbal products and processed foods. Such foods or their components may provide health benefits that go beyond basic nutrition.

Classification:

I. **Traditional nutraceuticals:-** natural food with no changes and intended to deliver various natural components that can provide health benefits (disease curing ability) apart from basic nutrition.

    1) Chemical constituents

        a) Phytochemicals: ascorbic acid, quercetin, luteolin, lutein, gallic acid, α-tocopherol, β-carotene and zeaxanthin

        b) Based on chemical class:

           • Carotenoids: β-carotene, lycopene

           • Dietary fibers: insoluble fiber, soluble fiber

           • Fatty acid: omega-3-fatty acid

           • Flavonoids: anthocyanidins, catechins

           • Phenols: caffeic acid, ferulic acid

           • Tannins: proanthocyanidins.

        c) Based on disease curing ability:

           • Anticancer: curcumin, capsaicin

           • Antioxidants: ascorbic acid, polyphenolics

           • Anti-inflammatory: curcumin, quercetin

           • Hypolipidemic: resveratrol, β-sitosterol.

        d) Dietary supplements: supplementing a diet with vitamin, mineral or herbals. Example- *Ginkgo biloba*is used as a supplement.

2) Probiotic microorganisms: They are friendly bacteria that promote healthy digestion and absorption. Example - *Lactobacillus acidophilus, L. lactis, L. brevis.*

3) Nutraceutical enzymes:

   - Plant source: pectinase, β-Amylase

   - Microbial source: Hemicellulase, Amyloglucosidase

   - Animal source: Pancreolipase, Chymotrypsin, α - Amylase.

4) Spices: cinnamon, clove, curcuma, saffron.

II. Non-traditional nutraceuticals:

1) Fortified nutraceuticals/Functional foods: orange juice fortified with calcium, cereals with added vitamins or minerals.

2) Recombinant nutraceuticals: Energyproviding foods such as bread, alcohol, fermented starch, yogurt, cheese, vinegar, and others which are produced with the help of biotechnology.

3) Nutricosmetics: it is a combination of nutraceuticals and cosmeceuticals. They are ingestible natural health products that enhance the function and appearance of an individual's skin, nails, and hair. For example - antioxidants, vitamins may be used in face cream.

   1. Name the different categories of nutraceutical products available in the market.

   A. Functional Food:

       i. Probiotics Fortified Food

       ii. Omega Fatty Acid Fortified Food

       iii. Branded Ionized Salt

       iv. Branded Wheat Flour Market

   B. Functional Beverages

       i. Fruit & Vegetable Juices

       ii. Dairy & Dairy Drinks

       iii. Non-carbonated Drinks

    iv. Herbal Tea, Sports Drinks and Energy Drinks

C. Dietary Supplements

    i. Proteins & Peptides

    ii. Vitamins & Minerals

    iii. Plant Extracts, Algal Extracts, Phytochemicals

    iv. Fatty Acids and Fibre

D. Personal care: skin care, hair care products with phytochemicals and antioxidants for health-promoting benefits.

2. Briefly explain the role of nutraceuticals in the treatment of peptic ulcers.

Peptic ulcer is a common disease in which the lining of the gastric mucosa gets damaged, and perforations lead to bleeding. The most common cause for peptic ulcers is due to infection by *H. Pylori.* The following phytoconstituents and herbs are used for the treatment of peptic ulcers as nutraceuticals,

a) Anthocyanin: it is a phenolic phytopigment that has significant preventive and curative antiulcer activity, acts by increasing the biosynthesis of mucopolysaccharides, thus improving the efficiency of the mucus barrier.

b) Silymarin is a flavonolignan complex present in *Silybum marianum.* The antiulcerogenic effect of silymarin is due to its inhibitory mechanism on the lipoxygenase pathway, avoiding leukotriene synthesis.

c) *Curcuma longa:* belongs to the Zingiberaceae family. Curcumin, which is the main phytoconstituent, exhibits anti-inflammatory and antioxidant properties by scavenging free radicals and regulates matrix metalloproteinase activity to exert an antiulcer effect.

d) *Camellia sinensis:* the phenolics compounds present exhibits strong antioxidant activity and also suppress various inflammatory modulators in the ulcer region.

e) Liquorice (roots of *Glycyrrhiza glabra):* belongs to the family Leguminosae. The main constituent of liquorice root is Glycyrrhizin. Acts by elevating the prostaglandin level and promotes mucus secretion from the stomach, thus increasing the life span of surface cells of the stomach and also exerts an anti-pepsin activity that ultimately leads to ulcer healing. It also shows antioxidant effect, which accelerates the ulcer healing process.

f) *Emblica officinalis:* belongs to the family Euphorbiaceae. It has anti-inflammatory and antioxidative properties, thus exhibiting healing effects on the gastric lining.

g) *Picrorhiza kurroa:* The most important active con-stituents of the roots and rhizomes of *P. kurroa* are the iridoid glycosides, picrosides I, II, and III, and kutkoside. Picroside I and kutkoside have exhibits gastroprotective properties, mainly through their antioxidative activity.

3. **Explain briefly the role of nutraceuticals in the treatment of gastritis.**

Gastritis indicates inflammation of the stomach lining and is mostly caused by infection of *Helicobacter pylori* and also due to NSAIDs. It can also be caused by irritation due to excessive alcohol, severe illness, autoimmune problems, radiation therapy, and Crohn's disease. Nutraceuticals in the form of phytochemicals and various herbs may benefit by affecting mucosal immune response, H^+/K^+ pump, histamine release from mast cells, build-up of mucus wall structure and regulating the prostaglandin, myeloperoxidase, and nitric oxide (NO) pathways.

Phenolic compounds available through a variety of fruit juices and edible plants such as strawberry, apple, tea etc. exhibits gastroprotective effects due to their ability in increasing the endogenous prostaglandins, reduction in histamine secretion, scavenging free radicals, thus preventing oxidative stress damage and gastric mucus stimulation. Amaranth seed extract, grape fruit seed extract and capsaicin, quercetin provide protection against gastritis. Quercetin can increase the activity of superoxide dismutase, which is an antioxidant enzyme and thus prevent lipid peroxidation to protect gastric mucosal cells against inflammation. Wogonin, a flavonoid obtained from a traditional Chinese herb (*Scutellaria radix*), has a strong anti-inflammatory action. It targets the arachidonic acid metabolism and inhibits the activation of 5-lipoxygenase (LOX) and COX-2.Curcumin is also known to inhibit the growth of *H. pylori* via inhibition of the shikimate pathway, which is necessary for the synthesis of aromatic amino acids in bacteria.

4. **Name the various nutraceuticals used and explain their role in the treatment of irritable bowel syndrome.**

Irritable bowel syndrome is a functional bowel disorder that is accompanied by abdominal pain or discomfort where the contents of the large intestine either move very fast or slow, leading to defecation disruption. The various forms of nutraceuticals that are used in the treatment of IBS are,

a) *Probiotics, prebiotics and synbiotics:*

- Probiotics are live microorganisms that, if administered in an adequate amount, provide a health benefit to the host. Probiotics may exert a beneficial effect on several pathogenetic pathways associated with IBS leading to restoration of altered gut microbiota by increasing the number of beneficial bacteria's (eg. *Lactobacilli*) and reducing the number of pathogens because of competition. This combined effect leads to a decrease of inflammation caused due to proliferation of pathogenic bacteria and restoration of normal colonic fermentation. *Saccharomyces cerevisiae* strains are taken as probiotics in IBS symptoms.

- Prebiotics: Prebiotics are defined as non-digestible, fermentable dietary components that exert beneficial effects on the host through the modulation of composition or activity of gut microbiota. Short-chain fructo-oligosaccharides improves digestive discomfort associated with patients with IBS.

- Synbiotics: Synbiotics are dietary supplements thatconsists of a combination of prebiotics and probiotics. It increases the levels and activity of beneficial microbes in the gut. *Bacillus coagulans* combined with fructo-oligosaccharides, a mixture of *Lactobacillus acidophilus, Lactobacillus helveticus and Bifidobacteria* in a medium enriched with phytoextracts, are various synbiotic preparations which relieves pain and bloating in patients with IBS.

b) *Plant extracts:*

- *Andrographis paniculata* (family - Acanthaceae): extract decreases elevated levels of cytokines mRNA expression, including TNF-α and IL-6, in patients with IBS.

- *Curcuma longa*(family – Zingiberaceae): extract which is rich in curcumin is known for its antioxidant, anti-inflammatory, anticancer properties and the ability to modulate gut microbiota.

c) *Phytoconstituents:*

- Boswellic acids are active components of *Boswellia serrata* (family - Burseraceae). They exhibit anti-inflammatory activity by inhibiting leukotriene and prostaglandin synthesis.

- Polyphenols: commonly present in dietary plants and fruits. Polyphenols cause the down-regulation of inflammatory mediators and NF-κβ. Example - resveratrol, epigallocatechin, curcumin, quercetin.

- Peppermint oil: The main component of peppermint oil is menthol; it has relaxant effects on gut smooth muscle.

d) Fibres: Psyllium or ispaghula are the seed husk of the plant *Plantago ovata*. The husk is the mucilaginous portion of the seed coat; it contains soluble, viscous and intermediate fermentable fibre, which has excellent water retention capacity. Upon absorbing water, it swells and forms a gelatinous mass which softens and increases the volume of stool which improves peristaltic movements leading to defecation.

5. **Give the biological source of chicory, mention its nutraceutical composition and other phytochemicals present and list out the health benefits of chicory.**

Biological source: *Cichorium intybus* is a perennial herb belonging to the family *Asteraceae*.

Nutraceutical composition: Carbohydrates, phenolic compounds (dicaffeoylquinic acids, chlorogenic acid), flavonoids, fatty acids (lauric acid, myristic acid, palmitic acid, linoleic acid, stearic acid), amino acids (Glutamine, glutamate, aspartate, asparagine, glycine, serin and arginine), sesquiterpene lactones, vitamins (B1, B2, B6 and C), and minerals (calcium, potassium, sodium and magnesium).

Phytoconstituents: the chief constituents are inulin (belongs to the group of non-digestible carbohydrates called fructans), sesquiterpene lactones (lactucin, lactucopicrin), guaianolide glycosides - chicoroisides B and C, caffeic acid derivatives (chicoric acid), fats, proteins, hydroxycoumarins, flavonoids (quercetin, catechin, anthocyanin), alkaloids, steroids, terpenoids, volatile oil (camphor, cymene and cuminal), vitamins (α-tocopherol), β-carotene and zeaxanthin.

Health benefits: different parts of the plants are used for various health benefitting purposes such as,

- Hepatoprotective
- Antidiabetic
- Antimicrobial
- Antioxidant
- Antimalarial

- Prevents osteoporosis
- Anthelmintic
- Radioprotective effect.

6. **Mention the biological source, constituents present and the health benefits of alfalfa.**

Synonym: Father of all foods

Biological source: *Medicago sativa*, belonging to the family Leguminosae.

Constituents:

- Alkaloids: asparagines, trigoneline, stachydrine
- Amino acids: medicanine, lysine, arginine, histidine, tyrosine, phenylalanine,
- Coumarins: myrsellinol, scopoletin, esculetin, 4-coumaric acid
- Enzymes: isoflavone reductase, vestitone, reductase, iminopeptidase
- Flavonoids: quercetin, myricetin, luteolin, apigenin
- Minerals: Ca, K, P, Mg, Fe, Zn, Cu, Se etc.
- Non-protein amino acids: l-canaverin
- Phenolic compounds: *p*-hydroxybenzoic acid, vanillic acid, *p*-coumaric acid, ferulic acids, sinapic acids, caffeic acid, naringenin, chlorogenic acid
- Phytoestrogens: coumestrol, genistein, diadzein
- Phytosterols: β-sitosterol, stigmasterol
- Volatile components: terpenes, limonene, linalool.

Health benefits:

- reduces cholesterol absorption and atherosclerotic plaque formation
- used in treatment of menopausal symptoms in women
- antidiabetic
- antimicrobial (gram-positive bacteria)
- Health beverages made from *M. sativa* improve digestive functions, maintain nutrition balance in the body, reduce cholesterol, improve bone health and delay ageing
- strong estrogenic activity is useful in the treatment of hormone-related cancers.

7. **Give the biological source of ginger and mention its role as a health food.**

Biological source: dried roots and rhizomes of *Zingiber officinale*, belonging to the family Zingiberaceae.

Constituents:

- Carbohydrates: starch
- Lipid: free fatty acid
- Oleoresin containing phenolic compounds
- Crude fiber
- Volatile oil:
    - Monoterpenoids: Geraniol, curcumene, β-phellandrene, 1,8-cineole, citral, borneol, linalool
    - Sesquiterpenoids: Zerumbone, α-zingiberene, β-sesquiphellandrene, zingiberol
- Non-volatile pungent principles: Gingerols, shogaols, paradols, zingerone
- Vitamins & minerals.

Health benefits:

- Gastrointestinal Disorders: it is mainly used in indigestion as it adsorbs and neutralizes certain toxins in the stomach and improves the production and secretion of bile from liver and gall bladder. Gastric complications like constipation, dyspepsia, bloating, gastritis, epigastric discomfort, gastric ulcer, indigestion, nausea, and vomiting can be effectively managed with ginger extract. Ginger has excellent antiemetic properties in motion sickness, cancer chemotherapy, postoperative nausea, and pregnancy associated vomiting.
- Useful in migraine
- Cardioprotective: Ginger has antiplatelet, ani-thrombotic and lipid-lowering properties.
- Anti-inflammatory: Ginger suppresses prostaglandin synthesis through the inhibition of cyclooxygenase (COX)-1 and COX-2 pathway. It also suppresses leukotriene biosynthesis by inhibiting 5-lipoxygenase (5-LOX).

- Chemo-preventive: gingerol causes a decrease in iNOS and TNF-α expression and increased caspases activation to exert its chemo-preventive action.

- Antioxidant: prevents tissue damage from oxidative stress.

- Antidiabetic: shows insulinotropic, insulin-sensitizing actions together with increasing glucose uptake via cell surface glucose transporter 4 (GLUT4) and repair of damaged carbohydrate and lipid metabolism.

- Ginger has also been used in veterinary medicine for various GI disorders of animals.

8. **Explain the use of fenugreek as a functional food.**

Biological source: consists of the dried ripe seed of *Trigonella foenum graecum*, belonging to the family Leguminosae.

Constituents:

- Fiber: rich in soluble dietary fiber.Contains saponins, hemicelluloses, mucilage, tannins and pectin. The fiber content of fenugreek seed extract helps to moderate metabolism of glucose in the digestive tract. Used as a source of natural antioxidants because of its fiber content. It has been estimated that 100 g of seeds can provide 65% of dietary fibers. One of the main soluble fibers of fenugreek seeds is galactomannan.

- Proteins: endosperm is rich in proteins such as lysine, globulin, albumin, histidine and lecithin

- Vitamins and minerals: contain phosphorus and sulphur and minerals like calcium, iron and zinc.

- Alkaloids: Trimethylamine, Neurin, Trigonelline, Choline, Gentianine

- Flavonoids: quercetin, rutin, vitexin

- Steroidal sapogenins: Yamogenin, diosgenin, smilagenin, sarsasapogenin

- Saponins: Graecunins, fenugrin B, fenugreekine

- Volatile oil: aroma component is a hemiterpenoid-γ-lactone.

Health benefits:

- Has good diaphoretic activity, generates sweat and thus help in cleansing toxins from the body.
- Performs lymphatic cleansing and thus removes toxic wastes, dead cells and trapped proteins from the body.
- Maintains mucus conditions of the body, mostly the lungs, by helping to clear congestion.
- Drinking fenugreek decoctions causes softening and dissolving of accumulated and hardened masses of cellular debris.
- Relieves cold, bronchial issues, influenza and asthma conditions.
- Causes lactation (increase in milk production for nursing mothers)
- Hypoglycemiceffect: stimulates insulin synthesis and secretion of insulin from the beta-pancreatic cells.
- Antioxidant: has radical scavenging activity and can prevent lipid peroxidation
- Chemo-preventive action: cancer-preventive effects could be due to increased apoptosis.
- Exhibits antibacterial and antifungal effect
- Increases pancreatic digestive enzymes and thus aids in digestion.

9. **Write a note on Garlic with special emphasis onits nutraceutical applications.**

Biological source: Garlic is the ripe bulb of *Allium sativum*, belonging to the family Liliaceae.

Constituents:

- Carbohydrates, dietary fiber
- Protein: amino acids like aspartic acid, serine, alanine, glycine
- Vitamins & minerals: minerals like phosphorous, calcium, selenium and germanium. Vitamins like riboflavin, thiamine, nicotinic acid and vitamin-C

- Sulphur-containing complexes: diallyl sulfide (DAS), diallylthiosulfate (allicin), S-allyl-l-cysteine sulfoxides (alliin)
- Volatile oil: citral, geraniol, linalool, α-phellandrene.

Health benefits:

- Antidiabetic: it is an effective dietary ingredient for lowering blood sugar. Garlic lowers blood sugar levels by decreasing the rate at which insulin is deactivated and degraded by the body and by increasing levels of circulating insulin.

- Anti-Inflammatory and Immunomodulatory Effects: reduces pro-inflammatory cytokines and interleukins. Also, antioxidant property helps in reducing oxidative stress-induced tissue damage and lipid peroxidation.

- Anticancer: People who consumes raw or cooked garlic in their diet are less likely prone to colon, stomach, breast and prostate cancers. Certain enzymes in cancerous tissues are totally inhibited by alliinase and other compounds contained in garlic.

- Cardioprotective: Garlic is considered good for the heart because it lowers cholesterol and triglycerides in the blood stream. Sulphur compounds of garlic, helps to smooth blood flow by preventing platelets from sticking together and clotting.

- Antimicrobial: effective against many bacteria, fungi, yeasts, and some viruses. The active principles of garlic interact with the nucleic acids of the virus, thus limiting its proliferation.

10. **Explain the nutraceutical importance of honey.**

    Biological source: Honey is a viscous sweet secretion obtained from the honeycomb of various species of bees, such as *Apis mellifera, Apis dorsata, Apis indica* and other species of *Apis*, belonging to family Apideae.

    Constituents:

    - Carbohydrates: The main sugars are the monosaccharides such as fructose and glucose. Disaccharides like sucrose and trisaccharide's like oligosaccharides are also present.

    - Proteins, enzymes and amino acids: The three main honey enzymes are

- diastase (amylase): converts starch or glycogen into smaller sugar units

- invertase (sucrase, α-glucosidase): converts sucrose into fructose and glucose

- glucose oxidase: converts hydrogen peroxide and gluconic acid from glucose

- Vitamins and minerals: Some of the vitamins found in honey include ascorbic acid, pantothenic acid, niacin and riboflavin. Minerals such as calcium, copper, iron, magnesium, manganese, phosphorus, potassium and zinc are present.

- Phenolics and flavonoids: Cinnamic acid, hydroxybenzoic acid, apigenin, pinocembrin, acacetin, abscisic acid and ferullic acid are present.

Health benefits:

- Antioxidant: Phenolics and flavonoids present in honey are mainly responsible for its antioxidant activity, and as such honey is useful in inflammation, cardiovascular diseases, ageing and neurological diseases, which are prone to oxidative stress.

- Antimicrobial: Honey has low pH and high osmolarity, and along with an array of various enzymes, it generates hydrogen peroxide to exert antimicrobial action.

- Cures cough in children's.

- Wound healing: antibacterial property and high viscous nature of honey help in maintaining a protective barrier and thus prevent infection and fastens wound healing.

- Improves fertility: since honey is rich in vitamins, iron, calcium and other minerals and amino acids, it can improve egg quality in women and improve general fertility in males.

- Improves gastric health: used for the prevention and treatments of gastro-intestinal disorders such as peptic ulcers, gastritis, gastroenteritis.

11. **Highlight the nutraceutical constituents of amla and state its health benefits.**

Synonym: Indian gooseberry

Biological source: it consists of dried and fresh fruits of the plant *Emblica officinalis* (*Phyllanthus emblica*), belonging to family Euphorbiaceae.

Constituents:

- Carbohydrates: Pectin, free sugars such as D-glucose, D-fructose, D-myo-inositol
- Vitamins & minerals: Calcium, phosphorous, iron, carotene, thiamine, riboflavin, and niacin. Rich in ascorbic acid
- Fatty acids: Linolenic, linoleic, oleic, stearic, palmitic and myristic acid
- Hydrolyzable Tannins: Emblicanin A and B, Punigluconin, Pedunculagin, Chebulinic acid, Chebulagic acid, Ellagotannin
- Alkaloids: Phyllantine, Phyllembein, Phyllantidine
- Phenolics: Quercetin, Kaempferol, gallic acid, ellagic acid
- Organic acid: Citric acid.

Health benefits:

- It can be used in fresh, dried or baked form. The dried fruit, seed, leaves, root, bark and flowers are frequently used for medicinal purposes and for their nutraceutical values
- Appetizer: The green fruits can be made into pickles which act as appetizers
- Antioxidant: it is a potential free radical scavenger due to the presence of ascorbic acid (Vitamin-C)
- Antidiabetic: controls blood sugar level by regulating the enzyme alanine transaminase, which is present in the liver
- Useful in respiratory disorders
    - Usefull in maintaining gastric health, relieves constipation
    - Relieves dental problems
    - Diuretic in nature.

12. **Write a note on ginseng with special emphasis onits nutraceutical values.**

Biological source: It consists of dried roots of *Panax ginseng*, belonging to the family Araliaceae.

Constituents:

- Saponins: rich in ginsenosides which are dammarane saponins. There are two types of dammarane saponins - the protopanaxatriol class and the protopanaxadiol class. Chikusetsusaponin, panxoside are also present
- Amino acids: rich in glutamine and arginine
- Polysaccharides: pectin
- Volatile oil: α-terpinolene, β-bisabolene, β-phellandrene, zingiberene, limonene
- Phenolics & flavonoids: catechin and kaempferol, gallic acid, vanillic acid
- Vitamins: thiamine, riboflavin, ascorbic acid, biotin
- Minerals: N, P, K, Ca, and Mg
- Non-saponin: gintonin.

Health benefits:

- Antioxidant activity
- Anti-inflammatory activity: ginsenosidescan suppress the NF-kB signalling pathway and inhibit the expression of macrophage-derived cytokines.
- Antimicrobial activity: effective against H1N1 influenza virus. Ginsenosides reduces virus-induced inflammatory cytokines.
- Cardioprotective: active components of ginseng canstimulate nitric oxide production, inhibit ROS production, increase blood circulation, and help in adjusting lipid profiles. It helps in maintaining proper blood circulation.
- Antiobesogenic effect: ginsenosides has the potential to increase energy expenditure by stimulating the adenosine monophosphate-activated kinase pathway and are capable of reducing energy intake.

- Antidiabetic: active metabolite of ginsenosides, can stimulate insulin secretion
- Used as a herbal dietary supplement to enhance sexual endurance, strength, and energy.
- Anticancer: ginsenosides inhibits tumour migration and metastasis.

13. Write a note on ashwagandha and its nutraceutical benefits

Synonym: Withania root, Clustered Wintercherry

Biological source: It consists of the dried roots and stems bases of *Withania somnifera*, belonging to family Solanaceae.

Constituents:
- Steroidal lactones: withanolides, withaferin A
- Alkaloids: withanine, somniferine, anaferine
- Phytosterols: stigmasterol, stigmasterol glucoside, beta-sitosterol
- Phenolics and flavonoids: syringic, p-coumaric, vanillic acid, catechin, kaempferol and naringenin.

Health benefits:
- Adaptogen: attenuate the negative effects of hyperglycaemia, glucose intolerance, increase in plasma corticosteroid levels, gastric ulcerations, male sexual dysfunction, cognitive deficits, immuno-suppression and mental depression
- acetylcholinesterase inhibitory activity of withania improves cognition
- Neuroprotective
- Antioxidant: decreases hepatic lipid peroxidation
- Increases haematopoiesis
- Anti-inflammatory activity: withanolides exhibits anti-inflammatory activity by inhibiting transcription factors NF-kappaB. Also causes selective COX-2 enzyme inhibition
- Antineoplastic and chemoprevention: possess cell-cycle disruption and antiangiogenic activity. Withania stimulates the production of cytotoxic T-lymphocytes and prevents tumour growth.
- Antibacterial and antifungal.

14. Highlight the nutraceutical potential of spirulina.

Biological source: Spirulina is a planktonic photosynthetic cyanobacterium. Spirulina is a blue-green algae found in sea water that consists of two most important species, namely, *Spirulina maxima* and *Spirulina platensis*, belonging to the family Oscillatoriacea.

Constituents:

- Carbohydrates: rhamnose, xylose, galactose, and glycogen are present in more quantity. Simple carbohydrates like glucose, fructose and sucrose arepresent in small quantities. Mesoinositol phosphate (carbohydrate), which is a good source of organic phosphorus and inositol, is abundantly present.

- Proteins: it has a very high protein content and is very effective in case of protein deficiency and malnutrition. It contains all the essential amino acids, but the quantity of sulphur amino acids is low.

- Lipids: It is the best source of gamma-linolenic acid after human milk. Other fatty acids present are linoleic acid and palmitic acid in large quantities

- Vitamins and minerals: extremely rich in Vitamin B12, B1, B2, vitamin C, vitamin D, and vitamin E. Rich in minerals like iron, calcium, chromium, copper, magnesium, manganese, phosphorus, potassium, sodium and zinc.

- Pigments: chlorophyll, phycocyanin and β-carotene

- Antioxidants: carotenoids such as astaxanthin

- Enzymes: rich in antioxidant enzyme superoxide dismutase enzyme.

Health benefits:

- Ideal food for sports person and pure vegetarians for their regular nutrient supply

- Prevents diabetes

- Reduces negative effects of stress

- Polysaccharides present have a stimulating effect on DNA repair mechanisms

- Phycocyanin stimulates WBC, thus improves immune health
- Vitamin C, E and various enzymes present make it a powerful antioxidant, retards ageing and promotes tissue repair
- Cardioprotective
- Act as anti-inflammatory
- Increases appetite and improves digestive functions.

15. Elucidate the potential interactions of hypericum

Hypericum perforatum belonging to the family Hypericaceae is commonly known as St. John's Wort. The chief constituents are hypericin, quercetin, hyperforin, chlorogenic acid etc. Hypericin is mainly responsible for the antidepressant effect of the plant. Hypericin acts by inhibiting the reuptake of neurotransmitters like 5-hydroxytryptamine and dopamine. The plant increases the activity of the CYP (cytochrome) family of enzymes which are mainly responsible for drug metabolism. It also activates P-gp efflux protein. When co-administered with other drugs or synthetic antidepressants drugs, due to the inducing effect on CYP enzymes and P-gp efflux proteins, the synthetic drug is rapidly metabolized and cannot reach the desired therapeutic plasma concentration, thus causing failure of therapy. Activation of P-gp efflux proteins shall cause rapid elimination of the drug reducing its efficacy.

- Interaction of St. John's Wort with immunosuppressants: patients who have undergone transplants are stabilized on cyclosporine (an immuno-suppressant drug). Such patients, if co-administered with hypericum, shows decreased plasma levels of cyclosporine due to its rapid pre-systemic metabolism and elimination. Such an effect shall cause the failure of therapy.
- Hypericum reduces the efficacy of oral contraceptives and increases the chances of pregnancy for women who are on such contraceptives if co-administered with hypericum. Such interaction also causes intermenstrual bleeding as a side effect.

- The statins simvastatin and atorvastatin are metabolized by the cytochrome family of enzymes (CYP34) and are also substrates for P-glycoprotein. Hence such drugs may not be able to exert their therapeutic action if co-administered with hypericum.

- Hypericum induces rapid clearance of warfarin due to inducing effect on P-gp efflux proteins and cytochrome family of enzymes resulting in decreased biological effect of warfarin.

16. Explain the herb-drug interactions associated with kava-kava.

Kava kava is a beverage or extracts prepared from the rhizome of the kava plant (*Piper methysticum*) belonging to the family Piperaceae. The major phytoconstituents present are kavalactones which are potent inhibitors of CYP 450 enzymes. Co-ingestion of kava with prescribed or over-the-counter medications or other herbal remedies that are metabolized by CYP enzymes might then result in elevated and potentially toxic plasma concentrations of the co-administered drugs or their metabolites. If CYP enzymes are inhibited, the drugs will not get metabolized, leading to increased absorption. Plasma concentration achieved will then go beyond the therapeutic window, causing adverse reactions.

- Kavalactones potentiate the effects of CNS depressants like benzodiazepines, barbiturates which can increase sleeping time, ultimately leading to coma

- Kava can potentiate sedation, intoxication and impairment of cognition and co-ordination when combined with alcohol

- Interaction with caffeine may cause Rhabdomyolysis

- Interaction between kava and levodopa causes dopamine–antagonism and thus may decrease the effect of levodopa.

17. Explain the herb-drug interactions associated with Ginkgo.

The leaves of Ginkgo are obtained from the dioecious tree *Ginkgo biloba,* belonging to the family Ginkgoaceae. Five diterpene lactones (ginkgolides A, B, C, J, M) are the major constituents present. *Gingko biloba* extract is used for the treatment of Alzheimer'sdisease. The constituents of Gingko have an inductive effect on the CYP enzyme family (cytochrome enzymes).

- *Ginkgo biloba* increases the metabolism of antiepileptic drugs such as valproic acid and phenytoin, both of which are substrates of CYP2C19, which may result in failure of epilepsy therapy.

- Oral co-administration of *Ginkgo biloba* can decrease the bioavailability of cyclosporinby decreasing its absorption.

- The active chemicals in gingko (ginkgolide, bilobalides etc.) have antiplatelet activity and are platelet-activating factor antagonists resulting in increased bleeding time on long term use, especially after any surgery. Thus, concurrent use of *Ginkgo biloba* with anticoagulant drugs such as warfarin or antiplatelet agents like aspirin can cause severe health risks leading to persistent bleeding

- *Ginkgo biloba* may also interact with antidepressants trazodone (serotonin antagonist and reuptake inhibitor), resulting in coma.

18. **Explain the drug interactions of Ginseng.**

Active components of various ginsengs are different, and thus wide variations exist among ginseng products. Co-administration of ginseng with other drugs may cause drug interactions. It was reported that it did not appear to have any effect on CYP enzymes, except for CYP2D6, which it may inhibit in the elderly. Ginseng extracts were demonstrated to modulate multidrug resistance efflux transporters in a number of cancer cell lines. Ginseng has been reported to interact with anticoagulant-antithrombotic drugs. Ginseng can decrease the anticoagulant effect of warfarin. Ginseng has a structure similar to steroids and may have additive effects with estrogens and corticoids. Thus, it is recommended that they should not be used together. It was also reported to decrease the effect of loop diuretics, antihypertensives, anxiolytics, alcohol, antidepressants, MAO inhibitors and mood stabilizers.

19. **Explain the interactions of Garlic with other drugs when taken together**

    Garlic, known as *Allium Sativum*, belongs to the family Liliaceae. Its active components are alliin and allicin. Can competitively inhibit CYP3A4 enzyme.

    - Combined use of fresh garlic homogenate with captopril shows synergistic effects in lowering the blood pressure, and also captopril can increase the antihyperlipidemic activity of garlic.

    - Garlic can increase the bioavailability and decrease the clearance and elimination rate of hydrochlothiazide when administered orally. Thus, garlic could be beneficial during the treatment of hypertension in patients with myocardial stress.

    - Active constituents of garlic, especially alliin and allicin, are antioxidant in nature and inhibits the production and release of mediators such as platelet activating factor, prostaglandins and thromboxane. Such an inhibitory effect on the production and release of one or more of these mediators may result in decrease in platelet functions. Thus, garlic inhibits platelet aggregation in a irreversible manner and may potentiate the effect of other platelet inhibitors such as prostacyclin, indomethacin, and warfarin.

    - Ingestion of garlic for 21 days increases the expression of duodenal P-gp efflux proteins, thus decreasing saquinavir (anti-viral drug) bioavailability.

20. **Write a note on drug interactions and adverse effects associated with ephedra.**

    Ephedra is also known as Ma Huang. Ephedra consists of the dried aerial parts of *Ephedra gerardiana,* belonging to the family Ephedraceae. Ephedra contains ephedrine alkaloids such as ephedrine and pseudoephedrine.

    - Screening tests for persons consuming drugs of abuse along with ephedra may be positive for amphetamines because of the similarity in structure between ephedrine alkaloids and amphetamines. The euphoric and stimulant effects of ephedrine are less intense but similar to those of amphetamines.

- Ephedra can also yield false-positive results for opiate screening.

- Numerous adverse effects have been attributed to the consumption of ephedra such as nervousness, anxiety, palpitations, headaches, nausea, hypertension, seizures, strokes, myocardial infarction, hyperthermia.

- Myocardial ischemia and infarction, dysrhythmias, and uncontrolled hypertension have been reported following consumption of ephedra.

- Cerebral vascular ischemia, intracranial haemorrhage, and central nervous system vasculitis can occur upon consumption of ephedra.

Ten marks category questions

21. Explain in detail the role of nutraceuticals in the management of diabetes with special emphasis on the various types of nutraceuticals used and their pharmacology.

Nutraceuticals used for the management of diabetes can be classified under the following categories,

A. Nutrients: Substances with established nutritional functions, such as vitamins, minerals, amino acids and fatty acids.

  a) Vitamin C: Vitamin C helps to control blood sugar levels and improves the patient's antioxidant status, thus reducing oxidative damages. Vitamin C helps to prevent the development of cataracts and nerve disorders in people with diabetes. It also inhibits protein glycosylation, which plays a critical role in the development of long-term complications associated with diabetes.

  b) Biotin: it is a member of the vitamin B complex and is necessary for metabolism. In diabetic patients, biotin stimulates liver glucokinase activity, increases insulin production, and enhances glucose uptake in muscle cells. Food sources of biotin include organ meats, soy, egg yolks and whole grains.

  c) Chromium: Chromium is a trace element that may be deficient in persons with diabetes. Chromium supplements may increase insulin sensitivity and improve glucose tolerance in patients with type II diabetes.

d) Magnesium: magnesium rich diet decreases the risk for diabetes. Scientific evidence indicates that there is an inverse correlation between magnesium intake and fasting insulin levels, suggesting an improvement in insulin sensitivity.

e) α- Lipoic Acid: it is a naturally occurring antioxidant with potent reactive oxygen species (ROS) scavenging activity. It protects the retina against ischemi are perfusion injuries. Ischemic injury to the retina is considered to be one of the major causes of visual loss and occurs in diabetic retinopathy. Alpha-Lipoic acid also increases insulin sensitivity.

f) Coenzyme Q10: depleted levels Coenzyme Q10 are seen in diabetic patients. Coenzyme Q10 improves insulin resistance, particularly in hypertensive patients.

B. Herbs and herbal extracts:

a. *Aegle marmelos* (Holy Fruit Tree): belongs to Rutaceae family. It acts by increasing utilization of glucose either by direct stimulation of glucose uptake or via the mediation of enhanced insulin secretion. The chief constituent of the drug is marmelosin A, B and C, which is a furocoumarin. Other coumarins are marmesin, psoralin and umbelliferone.

b. *Gymnema sylvestre* (Gurmar): belongs to Apocynaceae family. It increases secretion of insulin, promotes regeneration of islet cells, increases utilization of glucose, increases the activities of enzymes responsible for utilization of glucose by insulin-dependent pathways, decreases the activity of gluconeogenic enzymes and sorbitol dehydrogenase, and also causes inhibition of glucose absorption from intestine. Contains oleanane saponins (like gymnemic acid) and dammarane saponins (like gymnemasides). It also contains anthraquinone, flavones, flavonoids like epicatechin, apigenin, luteolin and kaempferol.

c. *Momordica charantia* (Bitter Gourd): It belongs to the Cucurbitaceae family. It may act by increasing hepatic glycogen. Vicine is the hypoglycaemic constituent present in the seeds.

d. *Trigonella foenum-graecum* (Fenugreek): It belongs to Papilionaceae family, widely cultivated in many parts of India. It increases glucose-induced insulin release through a direct effect on the isolated islets of Langerhans. Various extracts of different parts of this plant, fibres, proteins and saponins isolated from the seeds exhibit significant hypoglycaemic activity. The main alkaloid present is Trigonelline which exhibits good hypoglycaemic activity.

C. **Dietary supplements**: Agents derived from other sources (like pyruvate, chondroitin sulphate, steroid hormone precursors) also exhibits hypoglycaemic activity. Decrease in pyruvate dehydrogenase (PDH) enzyme activity may result in impaired insulin release from the islets cells of pancreas. Chondroitin sulphate has antioxidant properties and improves bone health in diabetic patients.

22. **Highlight the various nutraceuticals used as chemotherapeutics and chemoprevention agents, throw light on the pharmacology involved.**

The various types of nutraceuticals used in the treatment or prevention of cancer are,

a) **Vitamins and Minerals:** Vitamins A, C, E and trace elements like selenium have proven anticancer activities. They may act by modulating immune function or by exhibiting antioxidant properties, or by direct effects such as cell-to-cell interactions and modulation of enzyme activity. During chemotherapy, the patient's requirement of antioxidants increases; hence, supplementation with micronutrients can act as adjuvant therapy in cancer patients. Vitamin D also has good tumour prevention ability and can induce differentiation and apoptosis in some of the most predominant cancers. Antioxidants, vitamins and minerals are always protective against cancer as they protect DNA damage from the free radicals. Diets rich in fruits and vegetables are helpful in cancer protection. Antioxidants (vitamin A, E, C) obtained from such diet induce cell differentiation and growth inhibition to various degrees in human cancer cells through various complex pathways like inhibition of protein kinase C activity, prostaglandin E1-stimulated adenylate cyclase activity etc. Also, such vitamins and minerals synergistically increase the effects of various chemotherapeutic agents and hyperthermiatherapy thereby, acting as biological response modifiers. They alsoreduce the toxicity of several standard tumour therapeutic agents in normal cells.

b) Phytochemicals:

i. Epigallocatechin-3-gallate (EGCG): is the major catechin found in green tea *Camellia sinensis*, belonging to the family Theaceae. EGCG exhibits anticancer properties, which include anti-angiogenic activity by affecting the transcriptional expression of vascular endothelial growth factor, inhibiting tumour initiation and promotion by inhibiting signal transduction pathways, and inducing apoptosis in estrogen receptors in breast cancer cells and causing antimetastatic activity.

ii. Quercetin: it is a type of flavonoid obtained from various fruits and vegetables. The effects of quercetin are considered to be related to the induction of cell apoptosis through multiple mechanisms. Quercetin can inhibit melanoma growth, invasion, and metastatic potential of tumour cells. It also down regulates the expression of the heat shock protein known to influence apoptosis and growth inhibition of prostate tumours. Flavonoids are also free-radical scavengers and thus prevents oxidative stress, causes modulation of enzymatic activity, and inhibition of cellular proliferation. It also has anti-inflammatory activity. Some of the flavones act through topoisomerase II activity modulation. DNA topoisomerase II is an enzyme that catalyzes the double-strand breakage and re-joining of DNA and is vital forseveral cell functions. Quercetin significantly inhibits the expression of specific oncogenes and other genes, controlling various phases of the cell cycle.

iii. Genistein: it is isoflavone derived from soya beans (consists of the dried seed of *Glycine soja*, belonging to the family Papilionaceae) and is one of the major cancer preventive agents. Among isoflavones, the three major constituents which act as chemo-preventive and chemotherapeutic agents are genistein, diadzein, and glycitin. They are collectively grouped as phytoestrogens for their weak estrogen-like activity and bind preferentially to ER-β receptors. It inhibits the tyrosine kinase enzyme that is most often upregulated in cancer cells.

iv. Resveratrol: Resveratrol is the most important anticancer stilbene. It exhibits anti-proliferative activity due to its role as a phytoalexin. Inhibits growth by inhibiting hedgehog signalling pathway.

v. Curcumin: it is obtained from dried roots and rhizomes of *Curcuma longa* belonging to the family Zingiberaceae. It acts by inducing apoptosis in malignant cell lines by suppressing a number of key elements in cellular signalling pathways related to growth, differentiation and malignant formation. Inactivates NF-κ Band other metastatic genes. It also inhibits cell proliferation and induction of apoptosis.

c) Herbs and Spices:

i. Basil (*Ocimum basilicum*): exhibits antioxidant, antimutagenic, antitumorigenic, antiviral, and antibacterial properties. The major constituents are linalool, 1,8-cineole, estragole, and eugenol.

ii. Garlic (*Allium sativum*): belongs to the family Alliaceae. Allicin and Alliin are the major anticancer principles. It influences the genomic expression by affecting histone homeostasis. Inhibits histone deacetylase (HDAC). HDAC inhibitors induce cancer cell cycle arrest, causes differentiation and cell death, reduce angiogenesis and modulates immune response.

iii. Ginger (*Zingiber officinale*): belongs to the family Zingiberaceae. The principal constituents of ginger are gingerol, paradol, shogaol, and zingerone. It also has anti-inflammatory properties. Gingerol has been found to possess substantial antioxidant activity.

iv. *Aegle marmelos*: belongs to the family Rutaceae. Lupeol is the major anticancer compound present and is active against breast cancer, malignant lymphoma, and leukaemia. *Aegle marmelos* possesses significant antioxidant activity and reduces side effects of chemotherapy & radiotherapy.

23. Explain in detail the role of functional foods in the treatment and prevention of cardio-vascular disorders. Comment on their mechanism of action.

The various cardio-vascular disorders are hypertension, Coronary Artery Disease, Ischemia, Hypertrophy, Oxidative Stress, Vascular Injury etc. The various forms of functional foods used for the treatment and prevention of CV disorders are,

a) *Dietary plants (fruits and vegetables)*: fruits and vegetables are rich in phenolics and flavonoids,which exert a protective role in CV disorders. Several bioactive components in fruits and vegetables such as carotenoids, vitamin C, fibre, magnesium and potassium act synergistically or antagonistically to promote a holistic protective effect due to its antioxidant and anti-inflammatory effects.Vegetables like Broccoli and Soya (isoflavones), olive oil also has excellent cardio protective effects. Phenolics and flavonoids, owing to their anti-inflammatory and antioxidant properties, exert improved vascular functions. They exert their protective effects in CV diseases by inhibiting platelet aggregation, reducing oxidative stress, and decreasing LDL oxidation. Lowering blood cholesterol, inhibition of LDL oxidation, lowering blood homocysteine, and improved endothelial function are some of the primary effects of various phenolics present in fruits and vegetables. Soy protein contains isoflavone phytoestrogens, including genistein and daidzein. The isoflavone content is responsible for cholesterol-lowering effects. Isoflavones exert antiatherogenic effects through inhibition of LDL oxidation by binding to estrogen receptors. Soy also reduces systolic, diastolic, and mean blood pressure. Tomato is a major source of carotenoids; lycopene is the major constituent of tomato. It is a good natural antioxidant and has cardioprotective actions. Its antioxidant property contributes to the reduction of blood pressure. Lycopene inhibits the activity of an enzyme in cholesterol synthesis and thus prevents coronary heart disease.

b) *Vitamins*: Hypertensive patients are more vulnerable to oxidative stress as their internal antioxidant defence mechanism is very weak. The powerful antioxidant functions of vitamin C serve to reduce tissue damage due to oxidative stress and thus help to prevent endothelial damage. Vitamins like C and E improves endothelial function & arterial compliance and also has cholesterol-lowering effect. Vitamin D plays an important role in regulating calcium-phosphate homeostasis and also exerts immuno regulatory and anti-inflammatory effects. Vitamin D plays an important role as a cardiovascular protective agent by modulation of vascular tone, regulation of blood pressure, improving vascular smooth muscle cell functions and maintaining healthy endothelium.

c) *Herbs*:

- Garlic (*Allium sativum*): The sulphur compounds present are responsible for their dietary and medicinal functions. Cardiovascular protective effects of are due to the constituent allicin. Garlic inhibits platelet aggregation and enhances vasodilatation.

- Turmeric (*Curcuma longa*): Curcumin is the active component of turmeric. Curcumin is a potent polyphenolic antioxidant that reduces tissue damage caused due to oxidative stress. Curcumin also has anti-inflammatory properties and reduces LDL & triglycerides, inhibits platelet-derived growth factors, which is important in maintaining a healthy vascular structure.

- Green tea (*Camellia sinensis*): It decreases cholesterol level and LDL-HDL ratio. Tea contains Epigallocatechin-3-gallate, which helps to reduce blood pressure. The antioxidant flavonoids present in green tea improves vascular functioning and also has anti-inflammatory property.

24. Classify herb-drug interactions based on the mechanism of action and also add a detailed note on the various mechanistic pathways involved.

A. *Pharmacokinetic interactions:* such interactions are a result of altered absorption, metabolism, distribution and excretion of drugs leading to either potentiating or diminished activity of either of the component, leading to adverse reactions or failure of therapy as the case may be. Such interactions commonly occur in the liver, GIT and kidney.

a) *Induction and inhibition of metabolic enzymes:* Cytochrome P450 (CYP) is a generic term for a super-family of enzymes involved in the metabolism of xenobiotics and various other endogenous agents. The P450s are found mainly in the liver, intestines, kidneys, skin and lungs. Three main CYP families (CYP1,2, 3) are responsible for oxidative and reductive biotransformation of xenobiotics and other endogenous compounds in the body. Competitive CYP inhibition is dose-dependent and occurs when inhibitors compete with other substances for a particular enzyme. Non-competitive inhibition occurs when a substance either destroys or binds irreversibly to a CYP enzyme. In both instances, serum levels of those drugs chiefly metabolized by the affected enzyme, will become elevated due to poor metabolism of the drug, which causes increased plasma concentration of the drug beyond therapeutic levels, leading to toxicity and adverse reactions. On the other hand, many herbal medicines can induce CYP enzymes. Upon induction of CYP enzymes, metabolism shall be rapid and such phenomenon will reduce the oral bioavailability of the drug, and its systemic availability shall decrease, causing failure in therapy.

b) *Inhibition and induction of transport and efflux proteins:* efflux transporters are proteinaceous transporters localized in the cell membrane of all kinds of cells. Transporter proteins are associated with the transfer of some medicines from the intestinal lumen, through the biological barrier of the intestinal mucosa, into the systemic circulation and back again. P-gp also has a counter-transport activity, which means it can transport medicines from the blood back into the gastrointestinal tract, thereby reducing bioavailability. Transporters could be either carriers or pumps. Pumps are distinguished from carriers by the linkage of transport to an external source of energy. Examples of transporters in the intestine are P-glycoprotein (P-gp). The ATP-binding cassette (ABC) family of drug transporters plays an important role in the absorption, distribution and excretion of various medications. It is principally involved in the absorption and elimination of drugs from the intestine, liver, brain and kidneys. P-gp is a well-known member of the ABC transporter family, which is highly expressed in the apical membrane of several pharmacologically important epithelial barriers such as kidneys, liver, intestines and blood-brain barrier. Thus, co-administration of herbs with synthetic drugs can result in modulation of P-gp, which can affect oral bioavailability, biliary or renal clearance or brain uptake of drugs. Thus, the modulation of P-gp by herbal drugs may result in significant changes in the pharmacokinetics of prescription drugs and thus increase the risk of severe herb-drug interactions. Example - In cancer cells, P-gp is one of the transporters responsible for actively expelling chemotherapeutic drugs from cells, thereby decreasing intracellular concentrations and thus drug efficacy. As a result, identification of those substances that reduce P-gp expression can be administered safely with chemotherapeutic agents, but those agents which have inducing effects on P-gp cannot be used along with chemotherapeutic drugs.

c) *Alteration of gastrointestinal functions*: Herbal medicines can affect the bioavailability of synthetic drugs by altering the pH of the GI tract and other biochemical factors that affect the dissolution as well as the absorption of pH-dependent drugs. Also, the formation of complexes and chelates can further delay the absorption of synthetic drugs causing sub-normal plasma drug concentrations resulting in failure of therapy. Plants containing anthraquinone glycosides and soluble fibres of Guar gum and Psyllium can decrease GI transit time, thereby decreasing the drug absorption.

d) *Alteration in renal elimination*: Some herbal products are capable of interfering with renal functions, leading to the altered renal elimination of drugs. The inhibition of tubular secretion or reabsorption or interference with glomerular filtration are responsible for such types of interactions. On the other hand, certain herbal drugs can cause diuresis resulting in the quick elimination of drugs.

e) *Interactions with nutrients*: common in the case of interactions between iron and other minerals. Aluminium, calcium bicarbonate or magnesium trisilicate present in antacid preparations are known to reduce the extent of iron absorption owing to an alteration in gastric pH. Hence if any herbal ingredient is used along with conventional antacid, absorption of iron and its bioavailability shall be lower. This type of interaction is easily avoided by separating the intake of iron by at least 2 hours from the last dose of antacid.

B. *Pharmacodynamic interactions*: phytoconstituents and synthetic drugs may share a common receptor site which can either cause synergistic effects leading to pharmacodynamic toxicity or may cause antagonistic effects. Example - kava kava may have dopaminereceptor antagonist activity and therefore can interact with dopamine agonists (L-dopa), opposing their effect.

C. *Physiochemical interactions*: occurs when two substances come in contact and are either physically or chemically incompatible. This type of interaction can take place during the manufacture or administration of medicines and can affect both the rate and extent of absorption of one or both the drugs. Herbs with significant tannin content have the potential to be involved in physicochemical interactions with other medicines, both outside and within the body, because they form precipitates with proteins, nitrogenous bases, polysaccharides and some alkaloids and glycosides. Additionally, tannins will form complexes with metal ions such as iron, inhibiting their absorption.

25. Explain the different types of herb-food interactions, give suitable examples to justify your answer.

Pharmacokinetics or pharmacodynamic modifications of a herbal drug leading to altered absorption and bioavailability due to possible interaction with ingested food and nutrients is known as herb-food interaction. Such altered absorption of the herbal drug due to the presence of food or nutrients in GIT occurs due to the physical, chemical, physiological, or pathophysiological relationship between a drug and a nutrient. Food can affect the bioavailability of drugs by modification of drug absorption, metabolism, utilization, or excretion. Food can lead to either decreased bioavailability of a drug, which results in treatment failure or an increased bioavailability, which increases the possibility of adverse drug reactions.

Mechanisms of herb-food interaction.

a) *Alteration in gastric emptying*: Varying gastric emptying patterns have been identified for liquids, digestible solids, and non-digestible solids. Foods with high content of fat have been shown to decrease gastric emptying and hence delay the onset of pharmacological action of some drugs. Dietary protein can reduce GI motility and also stimulate pancreatic secretions. Protein and amino acids present in the ingested food are known to generate signals involved in the regulation of gastric and intestinal motility and pancreatic secretion.

b) *Complexation*: Complexation becomes a problem when an irreversible or an insoluble complex is formed between the drug and food present in GIT. In such cases, the proportion of the administered drug that forms complex become unavailable for absorption, resulting in reduction in bioavailability. The physicochemical characteristics of some diets could alter the pharmacokinetic properties of drugs by binding and transforming the drug into insoluble salts that are non-absorbable. For example – phenytoin (anti-epileptic drug) is bound by proteins present in food products, causing reduced phenytoin absorption and subsequent reduced bioavailability and treatment failure.

c) *Alteration in gastrointestinal pH*: After food ingestion, gastric pH is elevated as a result of the buffering and diluting effect of the food. This change in gastric pH greatly affects the absorption of many herbal drugs as the release profile, solubility, chemical stability, charge state and intestinal permeability of the drug depends on gastric pH. Furthermore, GI secretions like hydrochloric acid and pepsin released inresponse to the presence of food may lead to the degradation of drugs that are susceptible to chemical hydrolysis or oxidation, resulting in reduction in bioavailability. In some instances, GI secretion may increase bioavailability by enhancing dissolution of drugs.

d) *Enzyme induction/inhibition*: Nutrients present in food can either induce or inhibit cytochrome enzymes (CYP450) present in GIT. Induction of cytochrome enzyme shall lead to increased metabolism of herbal drugs resulting in decreased bioavailability. Whereas, inhibition of cytochrome enzymes shall cause slow metabolism leading to increased bioavailability which may cause adverse reactions, if the plasma concentration of the drug goes beyond the therapeutic window.

Example of herb-food interactions:

- Mango consumption increases the bioavailability of diclofenac due to inhibition of cytochrome family of enzymes.

- Black pepper, which contains Piperine, enhances the bioavailability of Fexofenadine drug due to inhibition of P-glycoprotein mediated cellular efflux.

- Green tea, which is rich in catechins, can influencethe activity of OATP (organic-anion-transporting polypeptides) transporters and also cause cytochrome P450 enzyme inhibition. OATPs are membrane influx transporters that regulate cellular uptake of a number of endogenous compounds and clinically important drugs.

Brain Teasers (for competitive exams)

1. **Who coined the word Nutraceutical?**

   The term nutraceutical was coined from "nutrition" and "pharmaceutical" in 1989 by Stephen DeFelice, founder and chairman of the *Foundation for Innovation in Medicine*

2. **Under which section classification of food has been prescribed by Food Safety Standard Act 2006?**

   Section 22, Chapter 4

3. **Under FSSA 2006, what do nutraceuticals include?**

   Vitamins, minerals, botanicals and herbal extracts

4. **Which is the regulating authority for nutraceuticals in India?**

   Food Safety Standards Act 2006

5. **Nutraceuticalswhich cover probiotics, antioxidants manufactured in liquids, tablets and capsules are known as?**

   Medical foods

6. **How many dietary minerals are required for maintaining human health?**

   20

7. **Cobalt is an essential component for?**

   Vitamin B12

8. **Mineral required for haemoglobin and collagen production?**

   Copper

9. **Vitamin K is useful in?**

   Blood clotting

10. **Which Vitamin responsible for the production of genetic material in cells?**

    Folic acid (Vitamin B12)

11. **Full form of PUFA?**

    Polyunsaturated fatty acids

12. **Sources of prebiotics?**

    Soybeans, inulin, raw oats, unrefined wheat and barley and yacon

13. **Foods that are manufactured by living microorganisms such as lactic acid bacteria, yeast and bacilli?**

    Probiotics

14. **Nutraceutical used as immunomodulators?**

    Ginseng

15. **The natural antioxidant present in tomato?**

    Lycopene

16. **Synonyms of fortified foodsare?**

    Designer foods

17. **Which nutraceutical principlesare present in Garlic?**

    sulphur-containing complexes such asdiallyl sulfide (DAS), diallylthiosulfate (allicin) and S-allyl-l-cysteine sulfoxides (alliin)

18. **Co-administration of *Ginkgo biloba* and warfarin causes?**

    Bleeding

19. **Piper increases the area under curve (AUC) of which drugs?**

    Phenytoin, Propranolol and Theophylline

20. **Spirulina (*Arthrospira Platensis*) is a type of?**

    Blue-green algae

21. **What is the botanical name of Kava-kava?**

    Piper methysticum (Piperaceae)

22. **Family of Honey (*Apis mellifera*)?**

    Apidae

23. **Phyllembin is anactive constituent of?**

   Amla (*Emblica officinalis*)

24. ***Momordica charantia*** **is predominantly used in which disease?**

   Diabetes mellitus

25. **Which family of enzymes is mainly responsible for drug metabolism?**

   Cytochrome P450 enzymes

Herbal Cosmetics, Herbal Excipients, Herbal Formulations

Two marks category questions

1. **Name the herbal raw materials used as extracts and oil for various hair care products.**

   Herbal oil:
   a) Amla – used as a hair oil
   b) Bhringraj – used as a hair tonic
   c) Coconut – used as hair oil and shampoo
   d) Eucalyptus – used as anti-dandruff
   e) Neem – used in hair oil, hair tonic
   f) Jatamansi – used as a hair tonic
   g) Lemon oil – used as a cleaning agent.

   Extract:
   a) Amla – shampoo
   b) Henna – used as a colourant
   c) Neem – used as hair conditioners
   d) Fenugreek – used as a hair tonic and anti-dandruff
   e) Ginko – used as shampoos
   f) Shikakai – used as shampoo and anti-dandruff.

2. **List out the advantages of herbal cosmetics.**
   - Compatible with all skin types
   - Low cost and affordability
   - Herbs offer more diversity of selection than synthetic compounds
   - Raw material readily available

- Lesser possibility of toxic or allergic reaction when compared to synthetic compounds.

3. **Give the classification of herbal cosmetics based on theiruse and application.**

   - Cosmetics for hair care: shampoos, hair oil, anti-dandruff, hair tonic, colourant, conditioners (heena, amla, onion etc.)

   - Cosmetics for skincare: anti-ageing creams, anti-acne creams, sun-screens, skin moisturisers, anti-wrinkle, anti-oxidant creams (amla, rosemary, ginseng etc.)

   - Cosmetics for eye care: eye gloss, eyeliners, eye shadows

   - Cosmetics as oils: used for both hair and skincare (jojoba oil, neem oil)

   - Fragrances and perfumes: oil extracted from flowers and fruits (sandalwood, oil from citrus fruits, mentha).

4. **Mention some mineral-based and some phytocompounds which are used as sun-screens or UV blockers.**

   Mineral-based: zinc oxide, titanium oxide and iron oxide

   Pytocompounds: silymarin, apigenin, ascorbic acid

5. **Name a major metabolic intermediate found in plants, animals and microbes which is used as skin antispetics.**

   Allantoin

6. **Define herbal syrup and mention its types and purpose.**

   The formulation prepared by incorporating concentrated herbal decoctions, infusions with a nearly saturated aqueous solution of sucrose or honey is known as syrup. Tinctures may also be used for making syrups. Alcohol may be added as a preservative. Generally, the syrup is made by mixing equal proportions of herbal infusion/decoction with aqueous sucrose or honey. They may be of two types, namely, medicated syrups containing medicinal plants (example – cinnamon syrup) and non-medicated syrups consisting of aromatic and flavouring plants (example – raspberry and orange syrup). Herbal syrups are used as a vehicle to deliver drugs which has a bitter taste or to pediatric patients. The main disadvantage of syrup is the problem of sugar crystallisation with time.

7. **Mention the advantages and disadvantages of natural excipients.**

Advantages:

a) No adverse effects, biodegradable, biocompatible (mostly carbohydrates) and non-toxic

b) Economical- easily affordable and easily available from nature.

Disadvantages:

a) Since they are obtained from nature, chances of microbial contamination are very high

b) Variation in quality due to changes in geographical and climatic conditions cannot be ignored

c) Dependability from nature slows down its production rate

d) Heavy metal contamination.

8. **Name some phytoconstituents which are used as colorants.**

Lawsone from Henna, curcumin from turmeric, betalins from beet, bixin and norbixin from annatto, lutein (carotenoids) from marigold and crocin from saffron.

9. **Name some phytoconstituents which are used as sweeteners.**
   - Terpenoids - stevioside, rebaudioside A, glycyrrhizin
   - Steroidal saponins - osladin, strogin, polypodoside A
   - Dihydrochalcones - glycyphyllin, trilobatin, naringin
   - Polyols - xylitol, erythritol
   - Proteins - thaumatin, miraculin, curculin.

10. **Name some phytoconstituents which are used as binders.**
    - Galactomannan
    - Tragacanthin and Bassorin
    - Fenugreek mucilage
    - Tamarind xyloglucan.

11. **Name some natural excipients which are used as diluents.**
    - Microcrystalline cellulose from conifer wood and cotton
    - Lactose from milk

- Gelatin
- Glucose from fruits
- Sucrose from cane.

12. Name two herbal excipients used as disintegrants.

Gums (gum karaya) and, Mucilage (*Plantago ovata*).

13. Name four herbal excipients used as preservatives.

Clove oil, neem oil, cumin seeds and turmeric.

14. Name four herbal excipients used as flavouring agents.

Menthol (from peppermint), d-limonene (orange), anethol (from anise) and limonene and cineol (from cardamon).

15. Name four herbal excipients used as perfumery agents.

Sandalwood oil (α-santalol & β-santalol), rosewood oil (linalool), eucalyptus oil (cineole), cedarwood oil.

Five marks category questions

16. Explain any five sources of fixed oils of herbal origin used as raw material in the preparation of herbal cosmetics.

Oils can dissolve fats and are widely used as an ingredient for the preparation of cosmetics. Oily materials reduce the evaporation of moisture from the skin and are used mainly to improve the feeling on use. The main components of oils and fats are triglycerides of fatty acids and glycerine. Oils are compounds that are liquid at room temperature, while fats are solid.

a) Olive oil: This oil is a fixed oil extracted from the fruits of *Olea europaea*, belonging to the family Oleaceae. The major constituents are triolein, tripalmitin, trilinolein, tristearate, monosterate, triarachidin, squalene, β-sitosterol and tocopherol. It is used as a skin and hair conditioner in cosmetics like lotions, shampoos etc.

b) Camellia oil: Camellia oil is obtained from the seeds of *Camellia japonica* belonging to the family Theacea. The constituent fatty acids in the oil are oleic acid (82-88%), saturated fatty acids such as palmitic acid (8-10%) and linoleic acid. It is used in cosmetic creams and milky lotions much the same way as olive oil. It is also used in hair oil.

c) Castor oil: This oil is obtained from the seeds of *Ricinus communis* belonging to the family Euphorbiaceae. The constituent fatty acid in the oil is ricinolic acid. It is used as an emollient in the preparation of lipstick, hair oils, creams and lotions.

d) Arachis Oil: This is a fixed oil obtained from the seeds of the *Arachis hypogea* belonging to the family Leguminoseae. It is used in the preparation of hair oils.

17. **Explain any three sources of waxes of herbal origin used as raw material in the preparation of herbal cosmetics.**

Waxes are a mix of esters, alcohols and fatty acids. It is primarily used as a thickening agent and also has protective qualities. It provides stability to skincare products and cosmetics and improves their viscosity and consistency, thus enabling them to stay on the skin surface for a prolonged time.

a) Jojoba oil: Jojoba oil is a liquid wax ester extracted from the seeds of the wild jojoba plant, *Simmondsia chinensis* and *Simmondsia californica* belonging to the family Euphorbiaceae. It is a desert plant. The main components are esters of unsaturated higher alcohols (11-eicosen-1-ol and 13-dococen-1-ol) and unsaturated fatty acids (11-eicosenoic acid and oleic acid). They were used in cosmetics as a moisturiser and as a carrier oil for exotic fragrances. Also used extensively in creams, milky lotions, lipsticks etc.

b) Carnauba wax: This hard, brittle wax is scraped from the leaves and leaf stems of wild or cultivated carnauba palms, *Copernicia cerifera* belonging to the family Palmae. Found predominantly in Brazil. It comprises esters of C20-C32 fatty acids, C28-C34 alcohols and large amounts of hydroxy acid esters. The main uses for carnauba wax are in stick cosmetics such as lipstick to improve the gloss and heat endurance

c) Candelilla wax: This wax is purified from the stems of the candelilla family of Euphorbiaceae plants (*Euphorbia cerifera, Euphorbia antisyphilitica*, and *Pedilanthus pavonis*). It is a desert plant. It is composed of approximately 30% C16-

C34 fatty-acid esters, and 45% hydrocarbons such as hentriacontane with approximately 25% free alcohols such as myricyl alcohol and resins. It is used mainly in stick products such as lipstick to improve gloss and heat endurance.

18. **Explain any four sources of gums of herbal origin used as raw material in the preparation of herbal cosmetics.**

Gums are pathological products produced by plants when they are injured, diseased or growing under unfavorable conditions. They are used as a thickening agent and helps to stabilise lotions and creams. Some of the commonly used gums of herbal origin are,

a) Xanthum gum: This gum is derived from the fermentation of the bacteria *Xanthomonas Campestris*. Xanthan gum is composed of chiefly D-glucosyl, D-mannosyl and D-glucosyluronic acid residues. Produces heat resistant cosmetic gels.

b) Guar gum: Guar gum is a seed gum produced from the powdered endosperm of the seeds of *Cyamopsis tetragonolobus* Linn belonging to the family Leguminosae. The water-soluble part of guar gum contains mainly a high molecular weight hydrocolloidal polysaccharide, galactomannan, which is commonly known as guaran. Guar gum is commonly used in lotion, cream, and ointment as an emulsifier, thickener, and stabiliser.

c) Acacia gum: it is a dried gummy exudation obtained from the stems and branches of *Acacia arabica*, belonging to the family Leguminosae. Acacia consists principally of arabin, which is a complex mixture of calcium, magnesium and potassium salts of arabic acid. In cosmetics, it is used as an emulsifier and thickening agent.

d) Almond gum: Almond gum is obtained from the tree *Prunus communis* (family: Rosaceae) in the form of a water-soluble gum that extrudes from the wounds on almond trees. The constitution of almond gum includes aldobionic acid, L-arabinose, L-galactose, D-mannose etc. In cosmetics, it is used as a gelling agent, stabiliser and emulsifier.

19. **Explain any five sources of bleaching agents of herbal origin used as raw material in the preparation of herbal cosmetics**

Bleaching agents or skin whitening agents are used in conditions of skin hyperpigmentation. They act by either inhibition of pigment synthesis or inhibition of enzyme tyrosinase which is the key enzyme involved in the synthesis of skin pigment melanin.

a) Gentisic acid (2,5-DHBA): it is a phenolic acid obtained from plants of *Gentiana* spp., *Citrus* spp., *Vitis vinifera*, *Pterocarpus santalinus*, *Helianthus tuberosus*, *Hibiscus rosa-sinensis* and *Olea europaea*. It improves skin whitening by inhibiting tyrosinase enzyme.

b) Arbutin: it is a glycoside, glycosylated hydroquinone extracted from the bearberry plant in the genus *Arctostaphylos*. Inhibits formation of skin pigment melanin.

c) Licorice extract: licorice extract is obtained from the root of *Glycyrrhia Glabra* belonging to the family Leguminosae. Improves hyperpigmentation by dispersing the melanin, inhibition of melanin biosynthesis and inhibition of cyclooxygenase activity, thereby decreasing free radical production. Glabridin, a polyphenolic flavonoid is mainly responsible for this skin whitening action

d) Mulberry extract: Mulberry extract is derived from the plant *Morus alba* belonging to the family Moraceae. It exhibits a skin lightening effect which may be due to inhibition of dopa oxidase activity of tyrosinase and superoxide scavenging activity.

e) Aloe vera extract: dried juice collected by incision from the bases of the leaves of various species of Aloe. *Aloe perryi, Aloe vera* or *Aloe barbadensis* and *Aloe ferox*, belonging to the family Liliaceae. The most important constituents of Aloes are the three isomers of Aloins, Barbaloin, β-barboloin and Isobarbaloin. Acts through reducing melanin aggregating effects leading to skin lightening via adrenergic receptor stimulation.

20. **Explain any five sources of antioxidants of herbal origin used as raw material in preparation of herbal cosmetics**

Antioxidants act by scavenging reactive oxygen species, which are formed as by-products of various metabolic pathways and can trigger oxidation reactions of the skin cells resulting in damage of skin cells.

a) Alpha-tocopherol: it is a pure phytoconstituent. Acts through glutathione pathway and inhibits lipid peroxidation.

b) Ascorbic acid: it is a pure phytoconstituent. Acts through scavenging of free radicals and regeneration of tocopherol.

c) Curcumin: it is a pure phytoconstituentobtained from rhizomes of *Curcuma longa*. Acts as a radical scavenger.

d) Quercetin: it is a pure phytoconstituent. Act as an iron chelator and maintain the balance of *in-vivo* antioxidant enzymes.

e) Carotenoids: it is a class of pure phytoconstituentssuch as β-carotene, lycopene and lutein. Prevents lipid peroxidation.

21. **Explain any five sources of protective agents of herbal origin used as raw material in the preparation of herbal cosmetics.**

Protective agents used in cosmetics are those entities that produce a coating on the skin mucosa, thus acting as an additional protective barrier, It is also involved in detoxifying mechanism either exogenously or endogenously and offers antioxidant protection and protection from ionising radiations as well.

a) Green Tea: Green Tea is made solely with the leaves of *Camellia sinensis* belonging to the family Theaceae. Green Tea is rich in polyphenols. It protects against direct damage to the cell and moderate's inflammation.

b) Turmeric: Consists of dried rhizomes of *Curcuma longa* belonging to the family Zingiberaceae. Curcumin is the main phytoconstituent present in turmeric. Scavenges reactive oxygen species, prevents lipid peroxidation and also act as a photo-protective agent.

c) Silymarin: It is flavonolignan obtained from the seeds of seeds *Silybum Marianum* (Family: Astraceae). It inhibits skin edema, prevents sunburn and cell apoptosis.

d) Resveratrol: It is polyphenolic phytoalexin belonging chemically to a class of compounds known as stilbenes, found largely in the skins of red grapes and root of *Polygonum cuspidatum*. It is a powerfull antioxidant and acts as a photo protective agent in cosmetics.

e) Avocado oil: Avocado is also known as *Persea americana*. Avocado oil comprises of Vitamin E, Vitamin D, β– carotene, protein, lecithin and essential fatty acids.

22. Write a brief note on herbal syrup.

Syrups are usually prepared by adding sucrose or honey to the herbal solution or decoction, followed by heating with continuous agitation and finally straining the resultant solution. Other sweetening agents may also be used. Sufficient purified water is then added and mixed well to yield a product of the desired consistency. Syrups should be made in quantities that can be consumed within a reasonable period of time. Syrups could be either medicated in nature containing a medicinally active herbal ingredient or maybe flavoured syrup used as a vehicle for administering bitter drugs. Syrups have a good soothing effect and demulcent effect as well and hence, are used frequently for cough preparations. The concentration of sugar in the syrup, according to IP, should be 66.7% w/w, and according to USP, it should be 85% w/v. At such a concentration, the osmotic pressure developed prevents the growth of microorganisms by disrupting the isotonic environment. If necessary, syrups may contain approved preservatives to prevent bacterial and mould growth. Syrups should be stored in dark glass bottles at a temperature not exceeding 30°C. Example – raspberry syrup, cherry syrup (used as a vehicle for delivery of antibiotics and cough preparations), glycyrrhiza syrup (masking agents for acidic drugs) and ginger syrup.

23. Write a brief note on herbal mixtures.

In many traditional systems of medicine, fine powders of herbal materials are taken directly by patients as a dosage form. Powders are prepared by grinding or pulverising dried herbal materials to suitable particle size. Crude drugs are processed and pulverised into various coarse or fine particle sizes. When used, they are suspended in warm water, ready for ingestion, or more commonly, they are packed into capsules or sachets. Commonly used for the treatment of GIT disorders.

24. Write a brief note on herbal tablets.

Tablets are solid preparations in which mono or polyherbal extract powder, plant powder or granule is blended with excipients and formed into a defined shape and size by compression. The different types of excipients or additives which may be added as per requirement are binders, glidants and lubricants to ensure efficient tableting. Disintegrants are added to ensure that the tablet releases its contents by disintegrating in the gut; sweeteners or flavouring agents are added to mask the bitter taste of the crude drugs and pigments to make uncoated tablets attractive in appearance. A coating may be applied to a tablet to mask the taste of the ingredients and make it smoother and easier to swallow. The coating protects the tablet from the acid secretionsof the stomach, allowing it to reach the target site like the small intestine or colon. Herbal tablets are normally designed for oral use with various herbal materials incorporated for a particular therapeutic effect using excipients. Herbal materials may be incorporated either by using finely powdered herbal materials or spray-dried plant extracts.

Steps involved in the preparation of herbal tablets

- Preliminary processing of crude drugs and weighing of the ingredients involved
- Mixing of herbal ingredients + excipients
- Conversion into granules (either by moist granulation or dry granulation)
- Compression of granules into tablets
- Coating of tablets (optional)

The stability of herbal tablets is very important as the shelf life of the tablet is largely affected by storage conditions and other environmental factors. The quality control parameters for tablets involve the study of their physical nature, content uniformity, friability, hardness and disintegration/dissolution testing. Example – asafoetida tablet for digestive disorders

25. Define and classify natural excipients.

According to WHO, the excipient is a non-active ingredient that has been adequately evaluated for safety and included in the delivery system too,

- Provide assistance during the process of development of a particular drug delivery system

- Improve the stability, bioavailability and patient acceptability
- Aid in the identification of the product
- Enhance any other attribute related to the safety and efficacy of the drug during storage and use.

I. *Classification based on source*

   a) Plant source: starch, peppermint, turmeric, cardamon, guar-gum

   b) Animal source: beeswax, cochineal, honey, gelatin, lanolin

   c) Mineral: bentonite, kaolin, talc, calamine, fullers earth

   d) Marine source: agar, carrageenan, alginic acid, laminarin.

II. *Classification based on application*

   a) Binders: acacia, tragacanth

   b) Fillers and diluents: dextrose and lactose

   c) Lubricants, Glidants, Disintegrants.

   d) Polishing Film formers and coatings agents

   e) Plasticisers & Colouring agents

   f) Suspending agents Preservatives& antioxidants

   g) Flavouring, Sweeteners & Taste improving agents.

   h) Printing inks & dispersing agents.

III. *Classification based on chemical nature*

   a) Carbohydrate: acacia, agar, cellulose

   b) Fixed oil: arachis oil, castor oil

   c) Fats: cocoa butter, palm oil

   d) Waxes: bees wax, carnauba wax

   e) Volatile oil: clove oil, cardamon oil, peppermint oil

   f) Resins: balsam tolu, asafoetida

   g) Proteins: gelatin, casein

   h) Enzymes: papain, diastase.

Ten marks category questions

26. Give a detailed account of various herbal raw materials used in oral products.

Oral products maintain oral hygiene by acting as antiplaque and anti-gingivitis. The antiplaque agents can be further subdivided as antiadhesives and antimicrobials. Some of the commonly used oral products which involve the use of herbals are,

a) Chewing stick: used both as antiplaque and anti-gingivitis. A small pencil-sized stick is chewed on one end until its edges are worn out and fibers exposed. The worn out and smashed end is used to clean the teeth. Various plants have been used in different parts of the world for this purpose. Arak (*Salvadora persica*) is mostly used in the middle east; lime tree (*S. aurantafolia*), and Neem (*Azadirachta indica*) in the Indian subcontinent. In the Middle East, "Miswak" is a traditional Arabic name used for any plant part that is used as a chewing stick. 'Datun' is the traditional name given to the chewing stick in the Indian subcontinent. Datun is made from neem (*Azadirachta indica*), mango (*Mangifera indica*), babul (*Acacia arabica*), guava (*Psidium guajava*) and pilu (*Salvadora persica*). Such plants exhibit potential antibacterial activity.

b) Tobacco based products: The use of tobacco-based products as a dentifrice is common in India. Lead to addiction as well.

c) Mouthwash: The use of mouthwashes made from the decoction of guava, pomegranate extracts, neem extracts, green tea, and cranberries juice have shown good efficacy in maintaining oral health. The addition of peppermint, cloves, aniseed, *aloe vera* gel and olive leaf enhances the antimicrobial activity of the toothpaste. Very effective in lowering plaque and gingivitis. All the above-mentioned plants are known to exhibit antibacterial effects inside the oral cavity and thus maintain a good oral health.

d) Charcoal: Used as a dentifrice, charcoal helps in maintaining the whiteness of teeth and prevents bad odour from the mouth.

Various medicinal plants have been extensively used in oral healthcare, namely, *Areca cathecu,* also known as betel nut, the fruit from the areca tree commonly known as "supari", reduce the incidence of caries and causes mechanical cleaning of teeth. *Phyllanthus emblica* is an excellent source of vitamin C and has anti-inflammatory and antibacterial properties. Used in the treatment of bleeding gums. *Ocimum tenuiflorum* (Tulsi) is widely used in all parts of India and is known to have strong antimicrobial properties towards *Streptococcus mutans*, one of the main organisms responsible for dental caries.

27. Give a detailed account of the involvement of herbal raw materials in skin care products.

The various types of skin care products, depending on their nature of use are,

a) *Anti-aging creams*: aging can occur either by age or may be induced by UV radiations from the sun. Skin aging is characterised by a reduction in the number of fibroblasts, collagen and elastin fibres which ultimately causes decay of the extracellular matrix. The balance between degradation and synthesis of collagen regulates skin aging process. Phytochemicals such as phenolic acids, saponins, alkaloids, and flavonoids have the property of inducing collagen synthesis and broadly utilised in the anti-aging topical cosmetics products. Herbals which are used as raw materials are,

- Ginseng: It consists of dried roots of *Panax ginseng*. Ginseng is incorporated as an anti-maturing component in facial creams. Prevents skin wrinkles and has antioxidative properties also.

- Carrot: Carrot is *Daucus carota*, belonging to the family Apiaceae. The main chemical constituents are β-carotene, and vitamin E, C, B and D. It promotes skin metabolism and increases skin immunity and antioxidative properties.

- Gingko: obtained from *Ginkgo biloba*, belonging to the family Ginkgoaceae. Contains flavonoids and terpenoids that enhance blood circulation and protect against skin damage. Gingko is known for its antioxidant, anti-inflammatory, and anti-aging activity.

b) *Skin moisturisers*: protects the natural moisture of the skin by preventing its evaporation.

- Coconut oil: obtained from *Cocos nucifera,* belonging to the family Arecaceae. Coconut oil has amazing skin smoothening and nourishing properties. Coconut oil has a sweet odour and excellent penetration capacity and thus act as a powerful moisturising agent. It replenishes the natural oils of the skin and gives a natural glow to the skin. It also helps in slowing down the aging effects and keeps the skin hydrated, thus giving it a soft feel.

- Jojoba oil: Jojoba oil is obtained from an American shrub called *Simmondsia chinensis*, belonging to the family Simmondsiaceae. Restores skin pH and also has antibacterial and anti-inflammatory properties.

c) *Anti-acne creams*: acne occurs when skin pores are blocked or infected. Some important herbals used in anti-acne creams are,

- Green Tea: It contains high concentrations of polyphenol antioxidants called catechins. Reduces sebum production and any associated inflammation.

d) *Anti-wrinkle creams*:

- Apricot: The vitamins A, C, and E, β-carotene and selenium contents of apricot show wrinkle prevention qualities.

e) *Sun-screen creams*: prevents tanning of skin due to denaturation of proteins and protects the skin from harmful UV radiations.

- *Cucurbita pepo* (Pumpkin): contains high levels of lipids such as linoleic acid. It also contains antioxidants such as tocopherols and phenolics. Exerts its sun-protective effects by protecting the peptide bonds of the skin proteins.

- Walnut: The extract is made from the fresh green shells of English walnut, *Juglans regia*. Its most important constitutent is juglone. Reacts with keratin proteins present in the skin to form sclerojuglonic compounds, which exhibits UV protection properties. It is used in the form of a scrub to diminish sun damage on the skin.

- Silymarin: Silymarin is obtained from the seeds of milk thistle (Silybum *marianum*). It is a flavonoid compound containing flavonolignans that prevents superoxide radical production. Several skin benefits of silymarin are antioxidant, sun damage protection, anti-acne, anti-inflammatory and skin brightening. Reduces UV light induced stress effects.

f) *Antioxidant skin creams*:

- Amla: *Emblica officinalis* with defensive antioxidant mechanisms.

- Rosemary: *Rosmarinus officinalis* is a rich source of phenolic compounds, and its properties are derived from its extracts and essential oil. Extracts of rosemary also contain several antioxidant and volatile components such as phenolic acids, flavonoids, and diterpenoids.

28. Give a detailed account of the involvement of herbal raw materials in hair care products.

Several formulations which are available as hair care products are shampoos, hair oil, hair conditioners and hair colourants. Such formulations are only for topical use and should have a local effect with no allergic reactions. Some of the herbals used as raw materials in hair care products are,

a) Brahmi: fresh or dried herbs of *Centella asiatica*, belonging to the family Umbelliferae. Brahmi contains essential oil, sterols, flavonol, glycoside and triterpenoid saponins. Delays aging of hair and promote hair growth.

b) Bhringraj: *Eclipta alba* Linn, belonging to the family Asteraceae. Bhringraj contains coumestans (wedelolactone and dimethyl wedelolactone), an alkaloid (ecliptine), glycosides (β-amyrin), triterpenic acid and steroids (ecalbasaponins). Used as a hair tonic.

c) Coconut: dried solid endosperm part of *Cocos nucifera*, belonging to the family Arecaceae. Oil of coconut fruit is used in different hair formulations, such as shampoos and hair oil. Coconut oil has a good saponification value so used in shampoos for hair care.

d) Eucalyptus: dried and fresh leaves of *Eucalyptus globules* belonging to the family Myrtaceae. Oil contains mainly cineole. Used for management of scruff and dandruff.

e) Henna: dried and fresh leaves of *Lawsonia inermis*, belonging to the family Lythraceae. Leaves mainly contain lawsone (quinone) and give a dark, intense orange colour. Henna leaves are used as hair colourants due to the chemical interaction of lawsone (thiol group) with that of keratin.

f) Onion: *Allium cepa*, belonging to the family Amaryllidaceae. Contains protein – Albumin. Other chemical constituents present are allin, allyl propyl disulfide, allicin and allyl sulfides. Helps in the maintenance of hair and enhances hair growth, also used for the treatment of baldness.

g) Lemon oil: oil extracted from the peels of *Citrus limonum*, belonging to the family Rutaceae. The lemon oil contains α-pinene, camphene, β-pinene, sabinene, myrcene, α-terpinene, linalool, β-bisabolene and limonene. Used as a hair cleaning agent.

29. What do you mean by herbal formulation? Give a brief account of various types of herbal formulations.

Herbal formulations are those types of dosage forms through which plant powder, extracts or bioactive phytoconstituents are delivered to a particular site of the body through various routes like oral, nasal, rectal, topical etc. Various types of herbal formulations are,

a) *Decoctions*: it is prepared by boiling the herb(s) in water for a certain period of time in order to extract the soluble constituents. Either a single herb or a mixture of herbs may be used. The water decoction of a mixture is the most common type of traditional herbal dosage form. Decoctions are normally carried out using harder plant parts (like barks and roots) that can withstand heat. Decoctions are normally intended for immediate use, ideally within a 24-hour period.

b) *Tinctures*: it is basically hydro-alcoholic extract of plant materials. Many plant constituents dissolve more easily in a hydro-alcoholic solvent when compared to water alone. Tinctures contain many structurally diverse compounds with varying polarities. The composition of hydro-alcoholic mixture depends upon the nature of the phytoconstituents to be extracted.

c) *Herbal glycerites*: Glycerites are made like tinctures, but in this case, hydro-alcoholic mixture is replaced by glycerine (used as extraction solvent). The concentration of glycerine should be at least 50 % to 60 % in the finished product for good stability. The shelf life is 6-24 months. However, glycerine should not be used for those drugs containing resins and gums. Glycerine is a good preservative for fresh plant juices, as it keeps the juice green and in suspension better than alcohol. This sort of preparation is called a '**succus**'. Glycerine is particularly good in making medicines for children and for soothing preparations intended for the throat and digestive tract or coughs.

Syrups: Syrups are viscous liquids containing sugars or other sweetening agents. They are prepared by dissolving, mixing, suspending or emulsifying herbal extracts or decoctions in a solution of honey, sucrose or other sweetening agents

a) *Herbal alcoholic beverages (bitters/wines)*: Herbal alcoholic beverages are normally ethanolic or hydro-ethanolic extracts of herbal materials.

b) *Oxymels*: An oxymel is a specialised sweet and sour herbal honey preparation used as a carrier for herbal infusions, decoctions, concentrates, tinctures, and other herbal extracts. Oxymels are used as a gargle or as a vehicle.

c) *Herbal capsules*: capsules are solid dosage forms where the active ingredient (drug) is enclosed in a practically tasteless gelatin shell. Drugs are normally more readily released from capsules compared to tablets. Capsules may help mask the unpleasant taste of its contents, and uniformity of dosage can be better achieved in capsules when compared to tablets.

d) *Herbal tablets*: Tablets are solid preparations in which mono or poly-herbal extract powder, plant powder or granule is blended with excipients and formed into a defined shape and size by compression. The different types of excipients or additives which may be added as per requirement are binders, glidants and lubricants to ensure efficient tableting.

e) *Herbal ointments*: Ointments are semi-solid preparations for application to the skin and mucous membrane. The base is usually anhydrous and immiscible with skin secretions. Ointments may be used as emollients or to apply suspended or dissolved medicaments to the skin. Herbal ointments normally have the plant material(s) either in finely sifted or in extract form incorporated into the base.

f) *Herbal balms*: it is basically an ointment used for massage into the skin for relief of body aches and pains. Contain herbal materials which provide a rubefacient effect on the skin and thus causes relief of pain.

g) *Herbal creams*: it is semi-solid emulsion that are mixtures of oil and water. Herbal creams normally contain the herbal material in either finely sifted form or incorporated as an extract.

h) *Medicated oils*: it is not essential oil but rather suspensions or solutions of herbal materials in an oily vehicle. Also known as macerated oils. These preparations are normally meant for external or topical use as liniments.

i) *Herbal pastes*: it is a topical paste and less greasy than ointments and may contain as much as 50 % powder dispersed in a fatty base.

j) *Herbal tea bags*: it comes as teabags packed with powdered herbal material. It can be consumed immediately by preparing a hot infusion.

k) *Aromatic waters*: it is a saturated water preparation of essential oils or other aromatic or volatile substances. Possess a characteristic odour of the essential oil used in the preparation.

l) *Plant powders*: consists of powders of herbal materials, which are taken directly by patients as a dosage form. Very fine homogenous powders are used in this case.

m) *Dry extract powders*: it is a solid preparation with a powdery consistency, obtained by evaporation of the solvent used for extraction. They may contain suitable added substances such as excipients, stabilisers and preservatives and are suitable for incorporation into a dry formulation like tablets or capsules.

n) *Granules*: it is a dried form of a liquid extract processed into spherical particles composed of agglomerations of smaller particles. Typically, granules can be reconstituted to form a herbal tea or infusion or may be compressed into a tablet or maybe filled into a capsule.

o) *Lozenges*: it is a solid dosage form that dissolves slowly in the mouth to provide local action in the oral cavity or the throat, such as cough drops or pastilles, but may also provide systemic action. Compressed lozenges are referred to as **"troches"**.

p) *Plasters and patches*: it contains dry or soft extract on pieces of fabric or plastic elastomer sheets in such a way as to adhere to the skin and attach to the backing. When applied topically to the skin, they deliver the active ingredients through the skin to the underlying tissues, used for relief of pain, backache or sore muscles.

q) *Inhalations*: intended for administration as aerosols to the bronchial tubes or lungs. Dry powders or liquid preparations can be administered through the inhalation route.

30. What do you mean by phytosomes? Explain in detail the working principle of phytosomes, highlight its properties and throw light on the available methods for characterisation of phytosomes. Name some commercially available phytosomes.

Phytosomes are also known as herbosomes. Phytosome is a novel drug delivery system where herbal drugs are loaded in vesicles, available in nano form. Phytosome provide an envelope, like coating around the phytoconstituent and keeps it safe from degradation by digestive secretion and bacteria in the gut. This is achieved by complexing standardised plant extracts or water-soluble phytoconstituents with phospholipids (phosphatidylcholine) in an aprotic solvent. Phosphatidyl, which is the tail part of phosphatidylcholine is lipophilic in nature, and the choline part, which is the round head, is hydrophilic in nature. The choline part attaches with the hydrophilic portion of the phytoconstituent. The choline and phosphatidyl parts are arranged in the form of a lipid bilayer, with the tail part facing each other to form a dense internal lipophilic layer, such type of complex results in better stability and bioavailability.

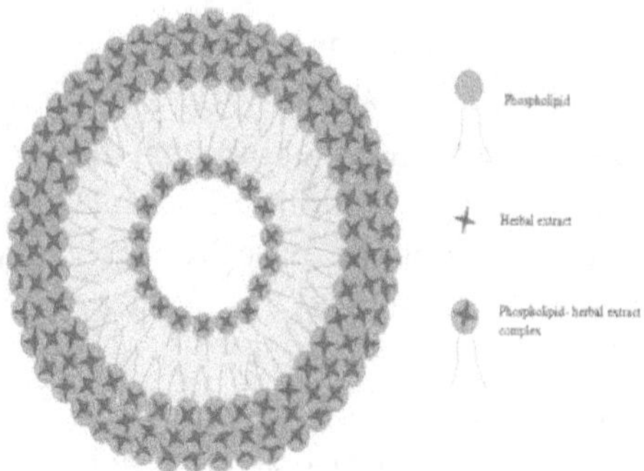

Phytosome

Properties of Phytosomes:

a) Phytosomes are a complex between phytoconstituents and natural phospholipids in a particular solvent.

b) Hydrogen bonding develops between the polar head of phospholipid and the polar groups of the phytoconstituents resulting in the formation of the complex.

c) When administered orally, increases the bioavailability of drugs. Particularly used for phenolics and flavonoids, which have a poor history of bioavailability.

d) Possess better pharmacokinetic properties when compared to traditional herbal formulations.

e) Have better stability.

f) Assures targeted delivery.

g) Reduces the dosage requirements of a drug

h) Provides better cutaneous drug absorption due to lipid bilayer.

i) Besides acting as a carrier, Phosphatidylcholine used in the preparation of phytosomes also acts as a hepatoprotective resulting in synergistic effect when hepatoprotective drugs are entrapped inside phytosomes.

j) Provides high drug entrapment.

Method of preparation: the phytosomal complex obtained by mixing phospholipid and phytoconstituentis mixed with ethanol and evaporated in a rotatory evaporator at a temperature of 60°C. A thin film forms around the flask during the process of evaporation. The film is hydrated by phosphate buffer at pH 7.4. Lipid layer is peeled off in the phosphate buffer solution, which is then sonicated to obtain a vesicular suspension.

Characterisation of phytosomes:

a) Differential scanning calorimetery: this technique is considered a useful tool to characterise the thermal behaviour of lipidic bilayers in the absence and presence of drugs

b) Scanning electron microscopy (SEM): used to determine the size and appearance of the particle

c) Transition electron microscopy (TEM): characterisesthe size of phytosomal vesicles

d) Drug entrapment and loading capacity:

Entrapment efficiency (%) =

$$\frac{\text{Wt.of total drug} - \text{wt.of free drug}}{\text{Wt.of total drug}} \times 100$$

e) Fourier transform infrared spectroscopy (FTIR) analysis: is done to check the structure as well as chemical stability of drug-phospholipid complex

f) Size analysis and zeta potential: to check the particle size and zeta size of phytosomal complex.

g) In-vivo studies: pharmacological studies based on animal models to evaluate the therapeutic efficacy of the drug.

Example –Phytosomes of Camellia sinensis or the extract of green tea, Grape seed phytosome, sinigrin phytosome, *Gingko biloba* phytosomes.

31. Give a detailed account of herbal excipients used as colourants

Colourants are used to add a distinctive appearance to a particular dosage form and thus enhance the aesthetic appearance of the dosage form leading to more patient acceptability. Plant pigments such as chlorophyll, carotenoids, flavonoids, anthraquinones, naphthoquinones, indole derivatives, oxyindole glycosides possess intense colours. Colourants are also known as chromogen and contain a chromophore group or auxochrome capable of absorbing light in the near UV regions and appears as coloured substance.

Ideal properties of natural colourants:

- Non-toxic and should not have any physiological effect
- Should have high stable colouring power
- Should remain unaffected by light, temperature, microbial contamination and upon longer storage
- Should remain unaffected by oxidising and reducing agents and changes to pH
- Compatible with the active ingredient of the drug
- Readily soluble in water
- Should not interfere with the assay of the active ingredient (drug)
- Easily available and economical

Some of the natural excipients used as colourants are,

Heena

Synonym: Mehendi, Lawsonia

Biological source: it consists of fresh and dried leaves of *Lawsonia inermis*, belonging to the family Lythraceae

Chemical constituents: the main colouring constituent is lawsone which is basically a naphthoquinone and is the degradation product of glucoside; hennoside A, B and C.

2-Hydroxy-1,4 - Napthaquinone

Other constituents are gallic acid, xanthone, tannins and mucins.

Uses: predominantly used as a hair dye, which imparts orange-red colour. Lawsone reacts with the skin and hair protein keratin and produces a strong stain. Also has hair conditioning, hair growth-promoting and anti-dandruff effect. Lawsone also has an antifungal and antibacterial effect.

Turmeric

Synonym: curcuma, haldi

Biological source: Turmeric is the dried rhizome of *Curcuma longa*, belonging to the family Zingiberaceae.

Chemical constituents: the major constituent is a yellow colouring principle known as curcuminoids, which comprises of curcumin (major ingredient, 60-70%), demethoxycurcumin and bis-demethoxy curcumin. Also contains volatile oil, namely, α- and β-pinene, camphene, limonene, linalool, isoborneol, camphor, eugenol, curdione, and curzerenone

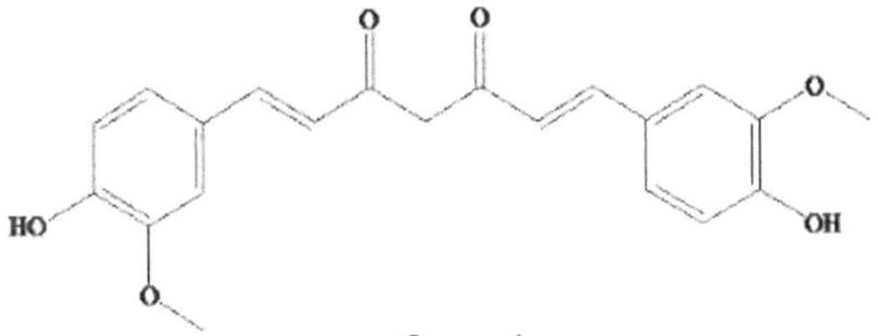

Curcumin

Uses: colouring agent, as an antibacterial in several herbal formulations, as spices etc.

Saffron

Synonym: Crocus

Biological source: Saffron is the dried stigma and styletops of *Crocus sativus*, belonging to family Iridaceae

Chemical constituents: Crocin is the chief colouring principle in Saffron. On hydrolysis, it yields digentiobiose and the carotenoid pigment crocetin. Saffron possesses a number of carotenoid-coloured compounds such as an ester of crocin, picrocrocin, crocetin, gentiobiose, lycopene, zeaxanthin, β-sitosterol, ursolic, oleanolic, palmitoleic, oleic acid etc.

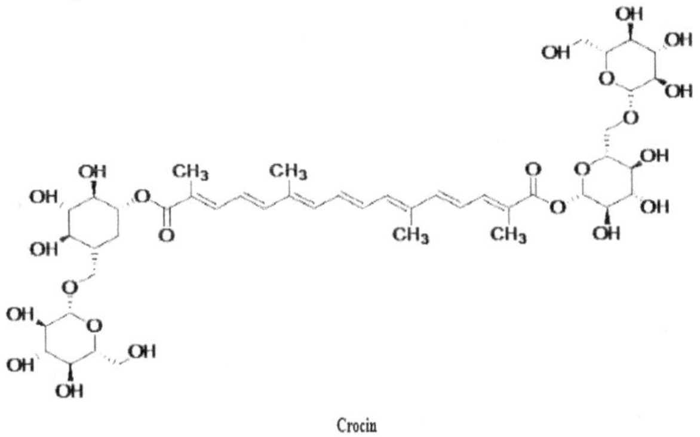

Crocin

Uses: apart from medicinal uses such as stomachic, fever, cold, it is mainly used as a colouring agent and in preparation of various herbal cosmetics.

32. Give a detailed account of herbal excipients used as sweeteners

Sweetening agents are those excipients that mask the taste of food, beverages and medications and make them sweet as well. In pharmaceutical industries, it is used in the preparation of liquid and oral dosage forms, providing a coating on tablets and pills and in preparation of vehicles such as syrup. Ideal properties of a sweetening agent are,

- Should be effective in small concentration
- Must be stable at a wide range of temperature
- Should have low-calorie output
- Should not exhibit batch to batch variations
- Should be compatible with the phytoconstituents involved in the herbal formulation.

Classification of natural sweeteners

A. Saccharides – sucrose, glucose, honey

B. Non-saccharides
- Terpenoids –steviosides, rebaudioside A, glycyrrhizin
- Steroidal saponins – osladin, strogin, polypodoside A
- Dihydrochalcones- glycyphyllin, trilobatin, naringin
- Polyols- xylitol, erythritol
- Proteins – thaumatin, miraculin, curculin

Stevia

Synonym: Honey leaf, Sweet leaf of Paraguay, Candy leaf

Biological source: obtained from the dried roots and leaves of plant *Stevia rebaudiana* belongs to the family Asteraceae

Chemical constituents: it is rich in terpenes and flavonoids. It consists of eight glycosides, namely, stevioside (300 times sweeter than sugar), steviolbioside, rebausiosides A-E, dulcoside A, pulcoside-A. Steviosides interact with a protein channel called

TRPM5, potentiating the signal from the sweet or bitter receptors, thus amplifying the taste sensation.

Uses: In addition to a natural sweetener, Stevia is also used in hypoglycaemic conditions, used as a diuretic, cardio tonic and tonic.

Liquorice

Synonym: Sweet liquorice

Biological source: Liquorice consists of peeled and unpeeled stolons and roots of *Glycyrrhiza glabra*, belonging to the family Leguminosae.

Chemical constituents: The chief constituent of liquorice root is Glycyrrhizin, which is 50 times sweeter than sucrose. Glycyrrhizin is found in the form of potassium and calcium salt of glycyrrhizic acid. Glycyrrhizinic acid is a triterpenoid saponin having an α-amyrine structure. It also contains sugar, starch, gum, protein, fat, resin, and asparagin.

Uses: Glycyrrhiza is widely used as a sweetening agent and also in the treatment of bronchitis, cold, flu, coughs, stress and tuberculosis.

33. Give a detailed account of herbal excipients used as binders

Binders are agents used to impart cohesiveness to the granules so that the tablet remains intact after compression as a result tablet of desired hardness can be produced. It also holds together all the components used in the dosage formulation. Binders are also used in the mixture to express plasticity or to increase the potential of binding between the formulated particles. Some of the ideal properties of binders are,

- physiologically inert,
- should impart adequate cohesion to the powders such that the adhesiveness is not lost upon subjecting the final product to storage at different temperature and humidity conditions.

Classification of binder,

    a) Solution binders: are applied by dissolving it in a solvent like water or alcohol. Example – cellulose, gelatin

    b) Dry binders: are added directly to the powder blend before subjecting to compression. Example – polyethylene glycol

Gum acacia

Synonym: Jaguar gum

Biological source: Guar gum is extracted from the seeds of the drought-tolerant plant *tetragonoloba cyamopsis*, belonging to the family *Leguminosae*.

Chemical constituents: composed of the complex polymer of galactose and mannose. The water-soluble part of guar gum contains mainly a high molecular weight hydrocolloidal polysaccharide, that is, galactomannan, commonly known as guaran

Uses: used as a colloid, binding agent, disintegrating agent in formulations of pills, emulsion stabiliser, used in peptic ulcer therapy, reduces blood sugar concentrations in diabetic and serum levels in hyperlipidaemia patients.

Tamarind seeds

Synonym: Imli

Biological source: obtained from the endosperm of the seed of *Tamarindus indica* Linn., belonging to family Leguminosae.

Chemical constituents: Tamarind xyloglucan (polysaccharides)

Uses: Tamarind gum is a polysaccharide made up of glucosyl: xylosyl: galactosyl having a ratio of 3: 2: 1. The polysaccharide derived from tamarind seeds is used by the wet granulation method to formulate matrix tablets to be specifically used for colon drug targeting.

Tragacanth

Synonym: Goat's thorn, gum dragon, gum tragacanth

Biological source: It is the air-dried gummy exudate, flowing naturally or obtained by incision, from the stems and branches of *Astra-galus gummifer* and other species of *Astragalus*, belonging to family Leguminosae.

Chemical constituents: Tragacanth comprises of two vital fractions, the water-soluble part is known as 'tragacanthin', and the water-insoluble part is known as 'bassorin'. Bassorin swells up in water to form a gel, whereas tragacanthin forms an instant colloidal solution.

Uses: It is used as a demulcent in cough and cold preparations and as an emollient in cosmetics. Tragacanth is also used as a thickening, suspending and emulsifying agent. Mucilage of tragacanth is used as a binding agent in tablets and also as an excipient in pills.

34. Give a detailed account of herbal excipients used as diluents

Diluents or fillers are pharmaceutical components that do not have any pharmacological effect but are necessary for pharmaceutical preparations. Diluents are chemically ineffective excipients, most of which are used in the formulation up to 80 percent to build up the necessary bulk of the dosage form. Diluents provide better tablet properties, such as improved cohesion or better flow.

Functions of diluents

- Provides better cohesion
- Facilitates direct compression
- Enhances flow
- Helps to adjust the weight of the tablet as per the capacity of the die.

Ideal properties of diluents,

a) Should not support microbiological growth in the formulation
b) Preferably should be colourless
c) Should not interfere with the dissolution and bioavalability of the tablet
d) Should be physiologically inert and non-interfering with other excipients
e) Should not allow segregation of granules or powder blend upon addition
f) Should permit size reduction, if required

Microcrystalline cellulose

Microcrystalline cellulose is partly depolymerised purified cellulose that exists as a smooth, white, odourless hygroscopic crystalline powder consisting of non-fibrous materials. The raw material used for the preparation of microcrystalline cellulose is pulp from fibrous plants such as conifer wood (conifers are a group of gymnosperm plants that produce seeds without fruit or flowers), even cotton (consists of epidermal trichomes of the seeds of cultivated species of *Gossypium herbaceurre*, belonging to the family Malvaceae) can also be used as one of the source of raw material. It is prepared by processing alpha cellulose produced as a pulp from fibrous plant material with mineral acids. It is commonly used as a binder, diluent and disintegrant.

Lactose

Lactose is one of the most frequently used diluents in many pharmaceutical formulations (including tablets, capsules and inhalers) due to its low price and biological acceptability. A disaccharide of lactose consisting of d-galactose and glucose fragments connected by a 1,4 glyosidic bond is typically isolated from milk.

Maize Starch

Synonym: Amylum

Biological source: Starch consists of polysaccharide granules obtained from the grains of maize- *Zea mays*; rice - *Oryza sativa*; or wheat -*Triticum aestivum*; belonging to family Gramineae.

Chemical constituents: Starch contains chemically two different polysaccharides, such as amylose (β-amylose) and amylopectin (α-amylose), in the proportion of 1:2. Amylose is water-soluble, and amylopectin is water insoluble

Uses: Starch is used as a nutritive, demulcent, protective, absorbent, disintegrating agent in pills and tablets and as a diluent in dry extracts of crude drug. Starch is also used in the preparation of dusting talcum powder for skin application. It is used as an antidote to iodine poisoning.

35. **Give a detailed account of herbal excipients used as viscosity builders.**

Viscosity modifiers are added to the aqueous mixture to increase its viscosity without changing other physical properties. It includes substances like thickeners, texturisers, gelation agents and stiffening agents. Viscosity modifiers convert liquids to gels, used in pastes or powders to prepare formulations according to the need of the end-users. Such modifications are required to make the formulation pourable and palatable.

Advantages of high viscosity in pharmaceutical formulations

- Inhibits crystal growth
- Improves physical stability
- Prevents conversion of metastable crystal to stable crystals
- Makes the formulation pourable
- Stays on the applied surface for a longer time and provides the desired smoothness

Disadvantages of high viscosity in pharmaceutical formulations

- Prevents dispersion upon sedimentation
- Slows absorption
- Creates operational difficulties during manufacturing
- Diffusion and rate of dissolution decreases

Ideal characteristics of viscosity builders,

a) Viscosity achieved should not change with temperature

b) Should not alter other physical properties like taste

c) Non-toxic and compatible with other excipients

d) Should produce a structured vehicle

e) Should be pourable

f) Should not alter the pH of the final formulation

Classification of natural excipients used as viscosity builders

a) Gums: acacia, tragacanth

b) Semisynthetic Cellulose derivatives: methylcellulose

c) Natural polymers: acacia, tragacanth, xanthan gum, carrageenan

d) Synthetic polymers: carbomer

e) Particulate association colloids: bentonite

Xanthan gum

Biological source: Xanthan is a microbial polysaccharide produced from *Xanthomonas compestris*.

Chemical constituents: Xanthan gum is composed of chiefly D-glucosyl, D-mannosyl and D-glucosyluronic acid residues.

Uses: depending on the rheological behaviour, it is widely used as a stabiliser, suspending agent in emulsion & paints and viscosity controller in abrasives and adhesives.

Gum acacia

Synonym: Jaguar gum

Biological source: Guar gum is extracted from the seeds of the drought-tolerant plant *tetragonoloba cyamopsis*, belonging to the family *Leguminosae*.

Chemical constituents: composed of the complex polymer of galactose and mannose. The water-soluble part of guar gum contains mainly a high molecular weight hydrocolloidal polysaccharide, that is, galactomannan, which is commonly known as guaran.

Uses: Used as a colloid, a binding agent, disintegrating agent in formulations of pills, emulsion stabiliser, used in peptic ulcer therapy, reduces blood sugar concentrations in diabetic and serum levels in hyperlipidaemia patients.

Carrageenan

Synonym: Chondrus extract, Irish moss extract

Biological source: It is a sulphated polysccharide obtained from the seaweed called Irish moss and the red algae *Chondrus crispus*, belonging to the family Gigartinaceae.

Chemical constituents: The main constituent is galactans which is known as carrageenan. Three major types of carrageenan are Kappa, Iota and Lamda-carrageenans.

Uses: Carrageenan is used as an emulsifying agent, stabilising agent, solubilising agent, and viscosity builder. Tooth paste, creams, lotions and other cosmetic products are prepared by using carrageenan. It is also used for inducing inflammation in animal models used for *in-vivo* anti-inflammatory screening of drugs.

36. Give a detailed account of herbal excipients used as disintegrants.

Disintegrating agents are those which induce break up or cause dispersion of the dosage form (tablet) upon coming in contact with the GI fluid. Disintegration results in the desegregation of the dosage form into its constituent particles, thus facilitating the release of the drug from the matrix, which in turn provides a larger surface area for dissolution. Dissolution follows disintegration. Disintegrants acts by swelling upon absorbing GI fluid or by effervescence, or by melting at body temperature. "Super-disintegrants" are newer substances with greater disintegrating efficiency and mechanical strength at a lower concentration. In contact with water, the super-disintegrants swell, hydrate, increase in volume,causing a disruptive change in the tablet. They also provide improved compressibility, compatibility and have no negative impact on the mechanical strength of formulations containing high-dose of drugs. Examples of herbal super-disintegrants – gums (gum karaya) andmucilage's (*Plantago ovata*).

Ideal characteristics:

a) Should cause quick disintegration at the desired site

b) Should have good hydration capacity

c) Should have poor gel formation capacity

d) Should not form complexes with drug

e) Should have good moulding and flow properties

Gum Karaya

Synonym: Indian Tragacanth

Biological source: it consists of dried exudate of the tree *Sterculia urens, Sterculia tragacanth* and other species of *Sterculia* belonging to the family Sterculeaceae.

Chemical constituents: Gum karaya is an acid polysaccharide. It is a chemical consisting of galactose sugars, rhamnosis and galactic acid.

Uses: used as a binder in the paper industry, disintegrant, thickening agent in dyes and also used as a bulk laxative.

Plantago ovata seed mucilage

Synonym: Ispaghula, Spongel seeds

Biological source: consists of dried seeds of *Plantago ovata*, belonging to family Plantaginaece

Chemical constituents: Ispaghula seeds contain about 10% mucilage which is present in the epidermis of testa. Mucilage consists of two complex polysaccharides, pentosan and aldobionic acid.

Uses: seeds are used as a demulcent and bulk laxative.

37. Give a detailed account of herbal excipients used as flavours.

They are also known as masking agents or bitter blockers. Flavour is a mixed sensation of smell, taste, touch and sight which involve a combination of physio-chemical and physiological actions that influence the perception of substances. Flavouring agents are used to mask the unacceptable taste of antibiotics, laxatives, antihistaminics in paediatric and geriatric formulations. Most commonly used for liquid dosage forms and chewable tablets.

Classification

a) Natural Flavours and Natural Flavouring Substances: Flavouring substances obtained from plant or animal raw materials, by physical (distillation), or enzymatic processes. They may be used in their natural state or in processed form but must not contain any artificial flavouring substances. Example - Mentha, Cinnamomum, Eucalyptus, Ginger Oil, Lemongrass oil, Peppermint Oil.

b) Natural identical flavouring agent: Flavouring substances that are chemically purified from an aromatic source or synthesized and have the same chemical composition as natural products. They cannot contain any artificial flavouring substances. Example - Methyl salicylate, alcohol, glycerin.

c) Artificial flavoring agents: These substances are chemically different and absent in natural products.These are typically produced by fractional distillation and through additional chemical manipulation of naturally sourced chemicals, crude oil or coal tar. Although they are chemically different, sensory characteristics are the same as natural ones. Example - cinnamaldehyde and benzaldehyde.

Peppermint oil

Synonym: Mint

Biological source: It is the oil obtained by the distillation of *Mentha piperita*, belonging to the family Labiatae.

Chemical constituents: The chief constituent of Peppermint oil is Menthol. Other minor constituents are isovalerate, menthone, cineol, inactive pinene and limonene.

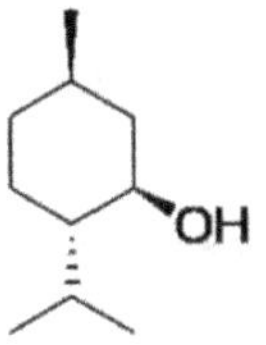

Menthol

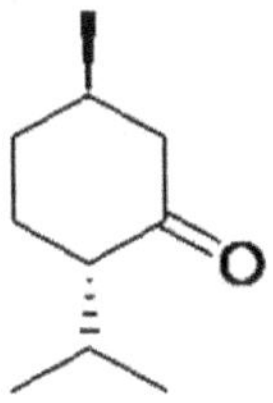

Menthone

Uses: apart from being a good flavouring agent, it is also used as a stimulant, stomachic, carminative.

Anise

Synonym: Sweet cumin

Biological source: Anise consists of dried ripe fruits of *Pimpinella anisum*, belonging to the family Umbelliferae.

Chemical constituents: The chief aromatic component of the essential oil is trans-anethole; also present are estragole, anisic acid, anisaldehyde, anise ketone, β-caryophylline and linalool. It consists of coumarins such as umbelliferone, scopoletin and flavonoid glycosides.

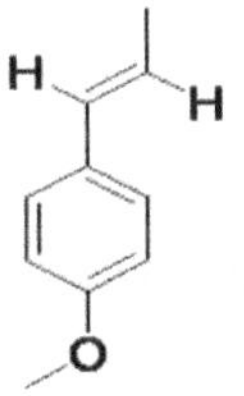

Anethole

Uses: apart from flavouring agent, it is also used as an expectorant, carminative, aromatic, antimicrobial, and antispasmodic.

Fennel

Synonym: Florence fennel

Biological source: Fennel consists of the dried ripe fruits of *Foeniculum vulgare,* belonging to the family Umbelliferae

Chemical constituents: The primary constituents of the volatile oil are 50 to 60% of anethole and fenchone. The oil of fennel has β-pinene, anisic acid, phellandrine, and anisic aldehyde.

Fenchone

Uses: used as stomachic, aromatic, diuretic, carminative, diaphoretic, as a digestive, pectoral, and flavouring agent.

38. Give a detailed account of herbal excipients used as perfumes.

Perfumes are generally used in the form of essential oil obtained by the process of distillation or other methods. Perfumery agents are used in improving the aesthetic value of the preparation. Essential oil, along with certain fixative agents such as benzyl alcohol, is used, which reduces the evaporation rate of the essential oil.

Sandalwood oil

Synonym: Chandan oil

Biological source: Sandalwood oil is obtained by distillation of sandalwood, *Santalum album,* belonging to the family Santalaceae.

Chemical constituents: The main odorous and medicinal principle is α-santalol (present in more quantity) and β-santalol.

Uses: Sandalwood oil is extensively used in perfumery preparations and also in soaps, face creams, and toilet powders.

Eucalyptus oil

Synonym: Stringy Bark Tree, Blue Gum Tree

Biological source: It is the essential oil obtained by the distillation of fresh leaves of *Eucalyptus globulus*, belonging to the family Myrtaceae.

Chemical constituents: Eucalyptus oil mainly contains 1,8-cineole, also known as eucalyptol. The other minor constituents are p-cymene, α-pinene.

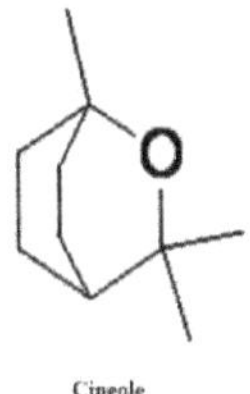

Uses: used as stimulant, antiseptic, flavouring agent, aromatic, deodorant, expectorant, antimicrobial, diuretic and antispasmodic.

Brain Teasers (for competitive exams)

1. **The appearance of dry and rough peeling of the skin is better known as?**

    Xerosis

2. **Cosmetic products containing herbal bioactive ingredients for improving health conditions of skin or hair is known as?**

    Cosmeceuticals

3. **Arbutin from bearberry is used as?**

    Skin whitening agent

4. **Crasonic acid from rosemary leaves used as?**

    Antioxidant

5. **Skin peeling in the form of small flakes from startum corneum of scalp causes?**

    Dandruff

6. **Synonym of soapnut (** *Sapindus mukorossi***)?**

   Ritha

7. **Type of alkaloid present in Tea?**

   Pseudoalkloids (Xanthine bases)

8. **Major Constituent of tea is?**

   Caffeine

9. **Phytochemical responsible for the colour of tea leaves?**

   Gallotannin acid

10. **Barbaloin, aloin and isobarbaloin is what type of glycoside?**

    C-glycosides

11. **Dabur Vatika hair oil is a marketed product of which crude drug?**

    Amla

12. **The main colouring agent of Henna is?**

    Lawsone

13. **Henna Hair colourant is more stable in?**

    Acidic medium (pH-5)

14. **Marine sources of natural excipients?**

    Alginic acid, Carrageenan, Agar and Laminarin

15. **Acceptable daily intake (ADI) of aspartame in ASU formulations**

    13.3mg/kg body weight

16. **Annatto is a type of?**

    Natural colourants

17. *Beta vulgaris* **(Beetroot) is a natural source of?**

    Betalains colourants

18. **Red dye from cochineal (insect) is due to?**

    Carminic acid

19. **The sweetness of Stevia, is due to?**

    Stevioside and rebaudoside (300 times sweeter than white sugar)

20. **Sources of Natural polymer binders are?**

Acacia gum, tragacanth and gelatin

21. **The common name of *Acacia concinnia*is is?**

Shikakai

22. **The Phospholipid required for the preparation of phytosomes?**

Phosphatidylcholine, Phosphatidylethanolamine or Phosphatidylserine

23. **Natural sun-screens or UV blockers?**

Mineral-based: zinc oxide, titanium oxide and iron oxide

Pytocompounds: silymarin, apigenin, ascorbic acid

24. **Major metabolic intermediate found in plants, animals and microbes, used as skin antispetics?**

Allantoin

25. **Organic Solvent required for dissolving phospholipids and drug extract to form a complex?**

Dioxane or acetone (Aprotic solvent)

26. **Name four herbal excipients used as preservatives**

Clove oil, neem oil, cumin seeds and turmeric

27. **What do you mean by oxymel?**

An oxymel is a specialised sweet and sour herbal honey preparation used as a carrier for herbal infusions, decoctions, concentrates, tinctures, and other herbal extracts

28. **Give some natural sources of super-disintegrants?**

Examples of herbal super-disintegrants – gums (gum karaya) and mucilage's (*Plantago ovata*).

Evaluation of Drugs, Patenting and Regulatory Requirements of Natural Products Regulatory Issues

Two marks category questions

1. **Define Patent?**

   A patent is a form of an intellectual property right granted by the Government to the applicant upon disclosing his invention (product or process) by virtue of which the patentee gets complete ownership of his invention and can legally prevent others from manufacturing, selling or using the said invention within a particular country for a specified time period. The invention must satisfy the patentability criteria for grant of patent. A patent is granted for a period of 20 years and is a territorial right that is valid within the country of grant.

2. **Mention the patentability criteria required for grant of patent to a particular invention.**

   a) Invention (product or process) must be new

   b) The invention must have an inventive step (non-obvious)

   c) The invention must have industrial applicability

   d) The invention should not fall under any of the provisions mentioned under Section 3 of the Indian Patents Act, which describes those inventions which are non-patentable

   e) The invention must not be related to Atomic energy (Section 4 of Indian Patents Act).

3. **Who grants an Indian patent, and how many patent offices are present in India?**

   The patent in India is granted by The Office of the Controller General of Patents, Designs and Trade Marks (CGPDTM),which is a subordinate office functioning under the Department of Industrial Policy and Promotion, Ministry of Commerce and Industry. There are four patent offices in India, Kolkata Patent Office (Head office), Delhi Patent Office, Mumbai Patent Office and Chennai Patent Office

4. Name the Act which governs the Indian patent system.

Indian Patents Act, 1970

5. List out the salient features of a patent.

a) A patent is granted for a term of 20 years

b) A patent can be sold and licensed

c) The patent has to be renewed every year upon payment of fees

d) A patent can be revoked by the High court, Appellate Board, Controller or Central Government on certain grounds

e) A patent is a territorial right, and hence, an Indian patent is valid only in India

f) A patent is granted for both product and process.

6. List out the various steps involved in the process of obtaining an Indian patent.

a) Applying for a patent in the prescribed format (Form 1, Form 2, Form 3 and Form 5 are mandatory) at the appropriate patent office by paying prescribed fees. The application can be submitted through both offline and online mode (e-filing).

b) Publication of the abstract of the application along with the details of the applicant in the official journal of the patent office after 18 months from the date of submission.

c) Examination of the application by a patent examiner upon submission of prescribed form (Form 18 asrequest for examination) and prescribed fee.

d) Generation of First examination report where the applicant is asked to submit a suitable reply against the objections raised by the concerned examiner.

e) Upon evaluating the reply filed by the applicant or his patent attorney, the final decision regarding the grant or rejection of the patent is taken by the Controller.

7. **Define IPR with examples.**

   Intellectual Property Rights are various types of legal rights that are offered to the creator of intellectual property for claiming ownership of the creation and preventing others from using the same without due authorization. Intellectual property is an original creation by a person using his own intellect ability or mind power. IPR provides legal options for taking ownership of such creations. Example – for innovation related to product or process – Patent is granted, for literary and artistic works – Copyright is granted, for creation like symbol or logo indicating a specific manufacturer or service provider – Trademark is granted, for agricultural or manufactured goods which owe their existence and quality due to its origin from a specific geographical location like Nagpur oranges, Mysore silk, Darjeeling tea etc. – Geographical Indication right is granted. All such rights, which are collectively known as IPR, are granted for a specific time period.

8. **Who is a breeder, and what are the breeders' rights as per the Plant Varieties and Farmers' Rights Act?**

   Breeder means a person or group of persons or a farmer or group of farmers or any institution which has bred, evolved or developed any variety. Exclusive rights are given to breeders to sell or produce for sell the propagating material, which is protected under the Act. Breeders can even import or export the protected variety and also can appoint licensee. Breeders are provided with a legal remedy in case there is any infringement case of the protected variety.

9. **What are the criteria's for registering a plant variety under the PPV&FR Act?**

   a) Novelty: a variety is considered to be novel if, before its registration for protection, the propagating or harvested material of such variety has not been sold or disposed of by the breeder anywhere in India (earlier than one year before filing for protection) or outside India (for trees or vines earlier than six years before filing for protection).

   b) Distinctiveness: the developed variety should be clearly distinguishable by at least one essential characteristics from any other variety whose existence is a matter of common knowledge in any country.

c) Uniformity: its essential characteristics should be sufficiently uniform during its propagation.

d) Stability: essential characteristics should remain unchanged even after repeated propagation.

10. Give the objectives of the Plant Varieties and Farmers' Rights Act (PPV&FR Act).

a) To establish an effective ecosystem for the protection of plant varieties and rights of farmers and breeders

b) To encourage the development of new plant varieties

c) To make available high quality seeds

d) To stimulate agricultural development in the country

11. Name the statutory bodies regulating ASU drugs.

- ASU-DCC
- ASU-DTAB
- Sub committee of Homeopathy and DTAB

12. Give an account of Schedule Z of Drugs & Cosmetics Act for ASU drugs.

Schedule Z deals with the requirements and guidelines for permission to manufacture ASU drugs for sale or to undertake clinical trials. Previously no clinical trials were required for ASU drugs, as such drugs are being used since ancient times. But the recent rejection of ASU drugs by western countries on issues related to quality and efficacy have forced the AYUSH ministry, which is the regulating body for ASU drugs, to impose Good Clinical Practice (GCP) guidelines on ASU drugs. As per schedule Z, it is mandatory for all ASU manufacturers to generate clinical trail data as per GCP guidelines. Such request for clinical trails has to be made prior to the start of manufacturing in form 24D. Institutional ethics committee approval is also required to begin the trials. Schedule Z has been opposed by the industries as such activity will increase the cost of the ASU drugs, the economic burden of which will be laid on the common man.

13. **Explain the importance of regulatory provisions for ASU drugs.**

- To lay down standards for the manufacture, sale and distribution of drugs
- To ensure the availability of standard drugs for people
- To ensure public health by protection from harmful and spurious substances

Five marks category questions

14. **Write a short note on bioprospecting.**

Bioprospecting is a systemic and strategic exploration of a region's biodiversity for the search and development of potential plant-derived organic compounds, genetic materials derived from plants & microorganisms and other bio-products along with various biochemical resources and utilizing them for the production of various pharmaceutical, agricultural, chemical entities which are of great social and commercial value. The different stages of bioprospecting are,

a) Scientific exploration of biodiversity for collection of samples (plants and microorganisms) from original habitat site.

b) Isolation, characterization and elucidation of various organic compounds and bacterial cultures.

c) Screening of samples for exploring their possible use in various fields like pharmaceutical, chemical industry, agricultural purposes etc. Those samples showing promising results are likely to be patented.

d) Product development and commercialization for revenue generation.

Advantages,

- Scientific usage of biodiversity without disrupting nature.
- Life saving drugs can be obtained by exploring such biodiversity, and with biotechnological interventions, for example – vincristine, vinblastine, taxol anticancer drugs are obtained from plant sources.

- Provides value addition to the available natural resources and ensures their conservation and sustainability.
- Bioprospecting is traditional knowledge-driven and hence provides a good opportunity for revenue generation for ethnic societies and some under developed countries.
- Improves quality of life for locals.

Disadvantages,

- Can lead to excessive exploitation of a regions biodiversity by developed countries, causing an imbalance in the local ecosystem.
- The ethnic community may be deprived of financial acknowledgement by the pharmaceutical companies.
- Patented products may be developed without giving due acknowledgement and profit-sharing to the ethnic community from whom the traditional knowledge was captured.

Different aspects of bioprospecting,

- Chemical prospecting: includes developments of drugs, pharmaceutical products, nutraceuticals, bio-pesticides etc.
- Gene prospecting: using genetic resources or a genetic pool for crop development, transgenic plant production, fermentation technology for production of various metabolites of medicinal interest.
- Bionic prospecting: developing new methods, designs, models, techniques based on natural biodiversity. Example-making engineered products from dolphin skin, using the sonic system of animals and insects in modern ultrasound imaging techniques etc.

15. Write a brief note on Bio-piracy.

Bioprospecting, when practised in an unethical manner fully committed for commercial benefits, neglecting the rights and benefits of the indigenous and ethnic community, constitutes a well-planned bio-piracy. Bio-piracy indicates unauthorized access of biological material and biochemical resources of a regions biodiversity and using them for commercial purposes along with obtaining patent rights by using indigenous knowledge belonging to a community, region of another country. Different categories of bio-piracy are,

a) Patent based bio-piracy: Patenting of various inventions related to biological resources or traditional knowledge that are obtained without adequate authorization and benefit-sharing from ethnic or indigenous communities of biodiversity-rich countries.

b) Non-patent bio-piracy: Produce commercialized non-patented products based on biological resources or traditional knowledge that have been unlawfully obtained from the indigenous people of a biodiversity rich country without giving any financial advantage to those groups who actually possessed the traditional knowledge.

c) Misappropriation: The unauthorized acquiring of biological resources or traditional knowledge from indigenous or local communities of another country without adequate benefit-sharing.

Demerits of Bio-piracy,

- Depletion of biodiversity

- Extinction threat for some endemic living organisms

- Privatization of traditional knowledge or indigenous genetic resources

- Economic disadvantage to the local indigenous community and to the country as well.

16. **What are the international laws and treaties made for preventing bio-piracy and protecting the biodiversity of a country?**

a) The Convention on Biological Diversity (CBD) and the World Trade Organization (WTO) Treaty on Trade-Related Aspects of Intellectual Property Rights (TRIPS). The CBD establishes the fact that a country shall have national rights over its biological resources and also commits member countries to conserve, develop and make it sustainable along with sharing benefits resulting from their use.

b) *Cartagena Protocol (2003):* The Cartagena Protocol on Biosafety to the CBD is an international agreement that aims to ensure the safe handling, transport and use of living modified organisms (LMOs) resulting from biotechnological interventions that may have adverse effects on biological diversity and human health as well.

c) *Nagoya Protocol (2010)*: It is an international agreement that aims at sharing the benefits arising from the utilization of genetic resources in a fair and equitable way, by appropriate access to genetic resources and by appropriate transfer of relevant technologies and also contributing to the conservation of biological diversity and its sustainable use.

d) *Cites 1972*: The Convention on International Trade in Endangered Species of Wild Fauna and Flora is an international agreement between governments. Its aim is to ensure that international trade in specimens of wild animals and plants does not threaten their survival.

17. Write a brief note on TKDL and mention its importance.

TKDL is Traditional Knowledge Digital Library and is a collaborative project between the Council of Scientific and Industrial Research, Ministry of Science & Technology and Department of AYUSH. Incidents of patenting Indian traditional knowledge in foreign countries lead to a deep need to develop a system for keeping vigilance related to such patents being filed anywhere in the world. In this regard, the cumulative efforts of Banaras Hindu University, Gujrat Ayurvedic University, National Institute of Ayurveda-Jaipur and Central Council for Research in Ayurveda and Siddha (CCRAS)-Delhi led to the development of an indigenously compiled digital database known as the Traditional Knowledge Digital Library (TKDL - http://www.tkdl.res.in/) containing information of more than 2 lakh traditional formulation prepared from medicinal plants and currently available in five international languages, namely, English, Japanese, French, German and Spanish. The formulations mentioned in the TKDL database are considered to be public property. Indian Government has entered into an agreement with patent offices of other countries that the TKDL database will be searched for finding any prior art for any patent filed which has relevance with traditional knowledge. Currently, the TKDL database is available to the patent offices of thirteen countries, namely, the Indian Patent Office, European Patent

Office, United State Patent & Trademark Office, Japan Patent Office, United Kingdom Patent Office etc.

Importance: TKDL serves as a public database of available traditional formulations of India. Information present in TKDL is treated to be in the public domain. Hence, such an available database shall prevent inventors from getting patents on traditional knowledge in foreign countries, as TKDL is accessed by foreign patent offices while examining a patent application.

18. Explain the patent revocation (cancellation) case of Curcuma.

In the year 1995, the United States awarded a US patent on wound healing properties of turmeric to the University of Mississippi Medical Center. The patent claimed the wound healing property of turmeric powder and its administration. There is astrong evidence in Indian culture regarding the use of turmeric in wound healing since ancient times. Based on this fact, the Council of Scientific and Industrial Research (CSIR) in 1996 challenged the patent and produced 32 references, some of which were more than 100 years old, in support of the fact that turmeric has been in use in Indian society and culture for its wound healing property since ancient times. The then CSIR Director-General Dr. R.A Mashelkar played a crucial role in this patent battle and fought till the patent got revoked or cancelled. Finally, the USPTO revoked the patent in 1997.

19. Explain the patent revocation case of Neem.

A European patent was granted by the European Patent Office for a fungicide derived from the seeds of the neem tree to the US Department of Agriculture and the multinational agribusiness corporation W. R. Grace in 1994. The patent was challenged in 1995 by the Indian Research Foundation for Science, Technology and Ecology (an environmentalist group) in association with the International Federation of Organic Agriculture Movements (IFOAM) and Magda Aelvoet, former green Member of the European Parliament. Several evidences were produced to support the fact that Indian farmers have been using neem-based formulations as fungicides since ancient times. A Pune based agrochemical company named Ajay Biotech produced relevant documents that it has been involved in making neem-based fungicide since 1980s. A signature campaign named 'Free the Free Tree' was also launched in India against this European patent. Neem is widely known as 'free tree' because it has numerous phytoconstituents for which neem-based products are widely used in medicine, cosmetics and agriculture. The patent was finally revoked by EPO in 2000.

20. **Mention in detail the constitution and functions of ASU DCC.**

ASU DCC is an advisory committee constituted by Central Government whose constitution is as follows,

a) Two nominated members by Central Government belonging to Department of AYUSH

b) One nominated member from each state government.

The Joint Secretary dealing with drugs in the Department of AYUSH and nominated by Central Government shall serve as the Chairman of ASU DCC, and the Adviser or Joint Adviser dealing with drugs in the Department of AYUSH and nominated by Central Government shall serve as the Member Secretary.

Functions:

a) The members shall hold office for 3 years and shall co-ordinate the meetings of ASU DTAB

b) May frame rules for regulating the conduct of the DCC

c) To advice the Central Government, DTAB and State Governments on matters arising out of the uniform administration of Drugs and Cosmetics act throughout the country.

21. **Explain the regulatory rules regarding the sale of ASU drugs.**

a) **Manufacturing in multiple premises**: separate license for each such manufacturing premises is required

b) **Licensing authorities**: State Government shall appoint licensing authorities.

c) **Application for license to manufacture ASU drugs**: An application for the grant or renewal of a license to manufacture andsale of any ASU drugs shall be made in Form 24-D to the Licensing Authority along with a fee of Rs. 1000.

For loan license, application should be made in Form 24E along with a fee of Rs. 600.

d) **Form of license to manufacture ASU drugs**: License as per Act shall be issued in Form 25-D and in Form 25-E for manufacturing under loan license. The license shall be issued within a period of three months from the date of receipt of the application.

e) The certificate of renewal of a license in Form 25-D shall be issued in Form 26-D. The certificate of renewal of a loan license in Form 25-E shall be issued in Form 26-E.

f) **Duration**: An original license in Form 25-D or a renewed license in Form 26-D, unless sooner suspended or cancelled, shall be valid for a period of five years from the date of its issue or renewed. An original loan license in Form 25-E or a renewed loan license in Form 26-E, unless sooner suspended or cancelled, shall be valid for a period of five years from the date of its issue or renewed.

g) **Conditions of license**: A license in Form 25-D shall be subjected to the maintenance of such conditions, namely, maintaining proper records of the details of manufacture, allowing an inspector appointed under the Act to enter any premises for discharging duties as per Act, shall maintain an inspection book in Form 35 to enable an inspector to record his impressions.

h) **Identification of raw materials**: Raw materials used in the preparation of ASU drugs shall be identified and tested. Genuineness, and records of such tests and methods shall be maintained.

Ten marks category questions

22. **Explain farmers right as per the Protection of Plant Varieties and Farmers' Rights Act, 2001.**

The Protection of Plant Varieties and Farmers' Rights Act (PPV&FR Act) seeks to address the rights of plant breeders and farmers on an equal footing. The Act protects the rights of farmers with respect to the contribution they make in conserving, improving and making Plant Genetic Resources (PGR) available for the development of new plant varieties.

a) *Access to seeds*: farmers can use their seeds (save, sow, exchange etc.), including those of protected varieties which they produce in the same manner as they would have done before the enactment of the said law. However, farmers are prohibited from selling any branded seeds of a variety protected under the Act.

b) *Benefit-sharing*: farmers, if providing plant genetic resources to breeders for developing new plant varieties, are entitled to receive a share of the revenue generated form the commercialization of such variety.

c) *Compensation*: if a registered seed sold to the farmer for cultivation fails to meet the expected agronomic performance even under recommended management conditions, the farmer is liable to receive compensation from the breeder.

d) Reasonable seed price: farmers have the right to access seeds of registered varieties at a reasonable and remunerative price, failing which the breeders exclusive right over that particular variety can be suspended, and compulsory licensing may be granted to some other entity for making the seeds available to the farmers at a reasonable price.

e) *Recognition and reward for activities related to conservation*: farmers are eligible to receive recognition and rewards from the national gene fund for outstanding activities related to conservation and providing excellent genetic resources resulting in crop improvement.

f) *Registration of farmers varieties*: the Act permits registration of farmers varieties even if it lacks novelty but has to satisfy the requirements of distinctiveness, uniformity and stability.

g) *Prior authorization for commercialization of essentially derived varieties*: when a source material of farmers variety is used by a breeder for developing an essentially derived variety, prior permission from the farmer is required before commercialization which shall empower the farmer to negotiate the benefit-sharing deal.

h) *Exemption from payment of registration fees*: farmers are exempted from payment of any fees for the registration of a plant variety or for availing any services rendered under the PPV&FR Act.

i) Protection from infringement: farmers may not be charged of infringement if they can prove that they were ignorant about any such existing variety whose rights have been infringed.

23. Explain in detail the WHO guidelines for the assessment of herbal drugs.

The basic objective of these guidelines for the assessment of herbal drugs is to,

- ensure quality, safety and efficacy of herbal drugs

- provide a basis for research based on which the quality, safety and efficacy of herbal drugs can be evaluated

- provide a common basis for which documents related to the registration of herbal drugs can be evaluated by regulatory agencies of any country.

Such assessment of data provides greater assurance to the consumers that the crude drugs used in the herbal preparations have been verified, properly identified and quantified per unit dose with complete documentation of safety and efficacy data prior to granting regulatory approvals for commercialization. More specifically, such assessment ensures that the contaminants and residue limits are well within acceptable limits. These guidelines for the assessment of herbal medicines are intended to facilitate the work of regulatory authorities, scientific bodies and industry in the development, assessment and registration of such products. The assessment should reflect the scientific knowledge gathered in that field. Such assessment could be the basis for future classification of herbal medicines in different parts of the world.

WHO guidelines for the assessment of herbal drugs are mentioned below. But these guidelines should be read along with the guidelines of GACP and GMP. The finished product starts its journey from the cultivation and collection of medicinal plants, goes through the manufacturing process and then gets its final shape of herbal drug, henceforth, the initial cultivation and collection practices must be done in accordance with WHO guidelines so that plants with adequate phytoconstituents and free from microbial contamination can be obtained. Good manufacturing practices as per WHO also ensures consistency of the finished product.

I. **Assessment of Quality:**

a) *Pharmaceutical assessment*: procedures and tests mentioned in the official monographs must be carried out to ascertain the quality, safety and efficacy of herbal drugs. Botanical identification through organoleptic and microscopic evaluation, physico-chemical evaluation, chemical evaluation, pharmacological evaluation etc. must be carried out as mentioned in the monographs. Manufacturing process of herbal drugs should be in accordance with Good Manufacturing Practices as prescribed by WHO.

b) *Crude plant materials*: exhaustive information regarding the correct botanical identity of the plant which includes its genus and species must be provided. A voucher specimen of all the plants used in the herbal preparation must be preserved for any future reference. Complete details regarding the plant parts used in the preparation, markers present in the preparation (preferably along with their content), the content of foreign matter, the microbial load should be well defined. The finished product must contain a batch number on its label. Wrong identification, improper usage of a plant part, excess microbial load, all such issues can severely affect the quality, safety and efficacy of herbal drugs. Assessment of quantity of the chemical constituents present in the finished product is very important as such chemical constituents are mainly responsible for exhibiting the biological activity, which can be adversely affected if such constituents are not present in optimal quantity and numbers.

c) *Plant preparations*: the manufacturing process of various plant preparations such as extracts, oils, tinctures, purified fractions etc., must be mentioned in detail. If any additional substance is added apart from the main crude drugs, then it should be properly disclosed. Well defined assay procedures must be described to estimate the quantity of markers present in the herbal preparations. The quantity of markers present is mainly responsible for the efficacy of the product. Either specific markers could be estimated, or a group of chemical constituents belonging to a specific class can be estimated (like – total phenolics, total alkaloids etc.).

d) *Finished products*: the manufacturing process and the composition of the finished products must be disclosed. An assay procedure for determining the quantity of markers or a specific class of phytochemicals present in the finished product must be described. Regulatory requirements of the finished product must be taken care of in light of WHO certifications.

II. **Assessment of Stability**: the physical and chemical stability of the finished product must be determined, and shelf life should be mentioned on the product label.

III. **Assessment of Safety**: Safety is a fundamental principle in the provision of herbal medicines and a vital parameter of quality control. The guidelines were developed with the view of expanding the monitoring of the safety of herbal medicines within the existing pharmacovigilance systems. In this regard, National pharmacovigilance systems should be closely linked to national drug regulatory systems. To function properly, a national safety monitoring programme for herbal medicines should be operated. The most common sources of information on adverse events and reactions to medicines are clinical trials and spontaneous reports. Reports must be sought from health-care professionals, from consumers, from manufacturers and from other sources such as National Poisons Centers, Drug information Centers, clinical trials and consumer organizations. Following data should be primarily reported, age, sex and a brief medical history of the consumer, details of suspected herbal product(s), administration details, the reason for use, adverse reaction data, all other medicines used (including self-medication) and risk factors (age, impaired renal function). As a basic rule, documentation of a long period of use should be taken into consideration when assessing safety. This means that, when there are no detailed toxicological studies, documented experience of long-term use without evidence of safety problems should form the basis of the risk assessment. Acute and long-term toxicity studies should be conducted as per WHO guidelines.

IV. **Assessment of efficacy**: A review of the relevant literature should be carried out for research studies. The pharmacological and clinical effects of the herbal materials and their constituents with therapeutic activity should be specified or described. The indication(s) for the use of the medicine should be specified. In the case of traditional medicines, the requirements for proof of efficacy should depend on the kind of use. As many herbal remedies consist of a combination of several herbal materials, and as experience regarding the use of traditional remedies is often based on combination products, assessment should differentiate between old and new combination products.

V. **Intended use**: Product labels and package inserts should be understandable to the consumer or patient. The package information should include all necessary information on the proper use of the product such as name of the product, quantitative list of herbal materials, dosage form (mentioned separately for adults and children's), use, mode of administration, duration of use, major adverse effects (if any), overdosage information, contraindications, warnings, precautions (during pregnancy and lactation), expiry date, lot number and holder of the marketing authorization.

VI. **What do you mean by stability testing? Explain stability testing of herbal drugs.**

Stability testing is a process by which the quality and efficacy of the herbal products can be ensured upon storage for a long period of time. The quality of herbal products varies with time due to the influence of temperature, humidity, light, oxygen etc. Henceforth, stability studies ensure that the herbal medicine remains suitable for consumption during shelf life when stored under prescribed conditions as mentioned on the label. Stability testing provides scientific evidence on how the quality of a drug substance or product varies with time under the influence of the above-mentioned environmental factors. There are two traditional approaches for determining shelf life,

a) Sample belonging to the same batch are stored at standard and accelerated storage conditions and tested periodically. Based on the results, the expiry date or shelf life can be calculated.

b) Samples from batches manufactured over a period of the last five years spanning six months are evaluated simultaneously. Based on the results, the expiry date or shelf life can be calculated.

Stability studies should be conducted on at least three primary batches. The primary batches should be of the same formulation as proposed for marketing. For new products, the batches should be manufactured to a minimum of pilot-scale by the same route and method, simulating the final process to be used for production. The stability studies should be conducted on the dosage form packaged in the container and the closure system proposed for marketing. Stability study should include testing of those attributes of the drug that are susceptible to changes during storage and are likely to influence the quality, safety, andefficacy. Such attributes are,

a) Physical parameters: colour, odour, taste etc.

b) Chemical parameters: colour reaction, pH value, weight variation, disintegration, bulk density, extractive values, estimation of the marker by suitable methods and chromatographic profiling. Herbal products contain various phytoconstituents, hence, the stability of each of the constituents is important in estimating the overall stability of the finished product. This can be achieved through a comparison of the product with standard chromatograms and other assay methods. Quantification of markers through HPLC, HPTLC, GC, LC-MS provides conclusive evidence on the overall stability of the product in termsof quality.

c) Biological parameters: suitable bioassay may be employed.

d) Microbiological parameters: microbial load as a function of time must be determined to assess the microbial stability (ability to resist microbial growth) of the finished product.

The frequency of testing at long term storage conditions should be every 6 months over the first and second year and annually thereafter. For accelerated storage conditions, frequency of 0, 3 and 6 months for a six-month study period is recommended. The recommended storage conditions for accelerated study are 40°C±2°C with a relative humidity of 75%±5%. The recommended storage conditions for long term are 30°C±2°C with a relative humidity of 60%±5%.

An Ayurvedic drug can be considered to be stable if "no significant change" occurs at any time of testing at accelerated storage conditions or at real-time storage conditions. Significant change" for a drug is defined as,

a) When there is a 20% change from the initial assay value (if analysed for its active compound).

b) When there is a 15% change from the initial assay value (if it is analysed for its active compound).

c) The appearance of new spots in TLC fingerprint or complete disappearance of the existing spot.

d) The physico-chemical parameters (moisture, ash, particle size) shall not vary beyond 25% of the initial value.

e) Failure to meet the acceptance criteria as per individual monographs or specifications.

f) Failure to meet acceptance criteria for appearance (Physical attributes).

24. Explain the patenting aspects of traditional knowledge and natural products with reference to the Indian Patents Act.

Patent applications related to traditional knowledge are governed by a set of different principles. The Receipt, Sorting & Distribution (RECS) section of the patent office shall screen all documents to identify all those applications which have any relevance with traditional knowledge. Such application shall be given the tag of 'Traditional Knowledge' by the RECS section so that the application can be examined by a dedicated group of examiners having expertise in handling inventions associated with traditional knowledge. The following golden principles must be taken into consideration for the assessment of novelty and inventive steps for evaluating any application having association with traditional knowledge. The below-mentioned category of inventions associated with traditional knowledge or natural products cannot be patented.

a) If the subject matter of the claims has relation to extracts of plant materials containing unidentified active ingredients (phytoconstituents), such type of claims cannot be considered to be novel when the use of such plants is already practiced in the society as a part of knowledge available through traditional knowledge.

b) Combining plants whose therapeutic effects are already known with other multiple plants, understood to have been known for treating the same disease, is considered to be an obvious invention lacking inventive step.

c) If an ingredient (plant material/active ingredient) is already known for the treatment of a particular disease, then it can be easily assumed that any combination product comprising of the said ingredient would be effective for the treatment of that particular disease.

d) Findings that reveal the optimum working ranges of traditionally known ingredients by routine experimentation is not considered to be inventive.

e) In the case where multiple ingredients are involved, and all are known to possess the same therapeutic effect according to the teachings of traditional knowledge, in such case taking out one particular ingredient from the composition cannot be undertaken as an invention.

f) If certain individual ingredients (plants or phytoconstituents) are already known for the treatment of a particular disease as per the teachings from TKDL, then it becomes obvious that a combination product comprising of such plants with other known plants having the same known therapeutic effect would likely be more effective than each of the medicinal plants when used separately. It is a clear representation of aggregation of properties causing an additive effect.

25. Mention in detail the constitution and functions of ASU DTAB.

The Ayurvedic Siddha Unani (ASU) DTAB was constituted by exercising the powers conferred by Section 33C of the Drugs and Cosmetics Act, 1940

The Ex-officio members are as follows,

i. The Director-General of Health Services, Government of India – Chairman

ii. The Drugs Controller General of India

iii. Joint Secretary handling Drug Control Cell, Department of AYUSH

iv. The Director, Central Drugs Laboratory, Kolkata

The nominated members are as follows,

v. Director Pharmacopoeial Laboratory of Indian Medicine, Ghaziabad

vi. One person from the Sub-Committee of pharmacognosy Ayurvedic Pharmacopoeia Committee

vii. Chairman of Indian Pharmacopoeia Commission

viii. Two persons from Ayurveda Pharmacopoeia Committee

ix. One person each from Unani and Siddha Pharmacopoeia Committee

x. One teacher in Dravyaguna&Bhaishajya Kalpana

xi. One teacher from ILMUL-ADVIA TAKLIS-WA-DAWASAZI

xii. One teacher in Gunapadam

xiii. One person each from Ayurvedic, Unani and Siddha drug industry

xiv. One practioners each from Ayurveda, Unani and Siddha system of medicine.

Functions:

a) The tenure of the board members is for three years

b) To advice the Government on technical matters arising out of the administration of this Act

c) To conduct by-laws to regulate the functioning of all activities

    d) Secretary (appointed by the Central Government) shall provide secretarial services

    e) The board may constitute sub-committees and appoint temporary members.

26. Explain in detail the various regulations of ASU drugs in India.

ASU drugs are covered under the Drugs & Cosmetics Act, 1940 by the insertion of chapter IVA in 1983. The regulations related to ASU drugs are well described in Chapters 1-IVA of Drugs and Cosmetics Act, 1940.

Chapter I: provides introductory information pertaining to the definition of ASU drugs, government analysts and inspector

Chapter II: provides provision for establishing the Drugs Technical Advisory Board, The Central Drugs Laboratory and The Drugs Consultative Committee for administering of the D&C Act pertaining to ASU drugs.

Chapter III: sets out guidelines for the import of drugs and cosmetics by laying down standards for determining the quality. ASU drugs are considered to be misbranded if it is coloured, coated or powdered to conceal any damage, if not labelled properly or if the label makes any false claims. Drugs are considered adulterated if it contains decomposed parts, poisonous or toxic substances and is processed under insanitary conditions. Cosmetics are considered to be misbranded if it contains unprescribed colours, improper labelling indicating any false claims. Cosmetics are considered spurious if it is an imitation product or imported under a false name and doesn't belong to original manufacturer.

Regulations regarding import of drugs &cosmetics:

    a) Drugs & cosmetics which are not of standard quality and is likely to be adulterated, misbranded or spurious cannot be imported.

    b) Patented medicine should have proper disclosures in the labelling.

    c) Any cosmetic containing any ingredient which may be harmful cannot be imported.

    d) Import of any prohibited drug.

e) If the Government is of the view that certain drug and cosmetics may contain such ingredients which may be harmful to humans or animals or may contain such ingredients which do not have any therapeutic justification for their presence, it can prohibit the import of such drugs and cosmetics in the public interest.

f) Government may classify certain drugs for whose importation license shall be required.

g) Prescribe methods of testing the quality of the drug or cosmetics.

h) Prescribe standardization methods, permissible colours, permissible limits of poisonous substances, specify those diseases which the imported drug must not claim to cure.

i) Regulate the places at which only those imports can arrive.

j) Mentioning of manufacturing and expiry date along with the scientific name of the plants involved in the products.

Penalties upon violation of the above regulations:

a) Importation of adulterated or spurious drugs and cosmetics shall attract imprisonment for 3 years and fine upto Rs. 5000. Re-conviction shall invite imprisonment for 5 years and fine upto Rs. 10000.

b) Importation of a drug or cosmetic other than the intended one shall attract imprisonment upto 6 months or fine upto Rs. 500 or both. Re-conviction shall invite imprisonment for one year and fine upto Rs. 1000.

c) Any drug or cosmetic imported in contravention of the provisions of any notification made under Section 10-A shall attract imprisonment for 3 years and a fine upto Rs. 5000.

Upon conviction, the disputed consignment shall be confiscated.

Chapter IV: indicates provisions for the manufacture, sale and distribution of drugs and cosmetics. Following regulations are prescribed,

I. Prohibition of manufacture and sale of certain drugs and cosmetics

    a) Manufacture, sell, exhibiting any drug or cosmetic which is not of standard quality, adulterated, misbranded or spurious is prohibited

    b) Any patented drug unless label includes adequate disclosures

    c) Any drug which is not in accordance with the license granted.

II. Prohibition of selling, stocking or exhibiting any drug which has been imported or manufactured in contravention to the said Act.

III. Persons who are not a manufacturer and involved in distribution must disclose to the inspector the details of the original manufacturer from whom the consignment was obtained.

IV. Every person holding a valid license must maintain all such records and register as required under the Act and must disclose the same to the concerned officers discharging their duties in accordance with the said Act.

V. Regarding pleas, claiming ignorance by the accused that he was ignorant of the nature, substance or quality of the drug in respect of which the offence has been committed shall not be accepted. Also, any drug or cosmetic shall not be considered to be adulterated or spurious or misbranded if the added substance was necessary from the manufacturing point of view and if considered fit for consumption. A person who is not the manufacturer shall not be liable for contravention if he is able to prove that the drug was acquired from a licensed manufacturer or dealer. Such a person also needs to prove that he under no circumstances could have known of any contraventions associated with the drug.

VI. Government shall appoint analysts and inspectors under the provisions of the said Act. The powers of analysts and inspectors are well prescribed.

VII. Persons are bound to disclose the place where drugs or cosmetics are manufactured or kept.

VIII. Any person shall, upon application in the prescribed manner and on payment of the prescribed fee, be entitled to submit for test or analysis to a Government Analyst any drug or cosmetic purchased by him.

IX. If the Central Government is satisfied that the use of any drug or cosmetic is likely to involve any risk to human beings or animals or that any drug does not have the therapeutic value claimed or contains ingredients for which there is no therapeutic justification, Government then in the public interest can prohibit the manufacture, sale or distribution of such drug or cosmetic.

X. If the Central Government is satisfied that a drug is essential to meet the requirements of an emergency arising due to epidemic or natural calamities and that in the public interest, Government may regulate or restrict the manufacture, sale or distribution of such drug.

XI. Penalty arising out of any contravention may comprise of 7-10 years of imprisonment and/or a fine between 2-3 lakhs.

Chapter IVA: Provisions Relating to ASU Drugs, Lays down the constitution and functions of ASU-DTAB and ASU DCC. Following regulations are prescribed,

a) Regulation of manufacture for sale of ASU drugs: No person shall manufacture for sale or for distribution any ASU drug except in accordance with such standards if any, as may be prescribed in relation to that drug.

b) Prohibition of manufacture and sale of certain ASU drugs which are misbranded, adulterated or spurious. If patented, adequate disclosers on the label should be present.

c) Manufacture for sale or for distribution, any ASU drug, except under, and in accordance with the conditions of the license issued for such purpose.

d) These provisions shall not be applicable to Vaidyas and Hakims, who prepare drugs for their own patients.

e) If the Central Government is satisfied on the basis of any evidence or other material available before it that the use of any ASU drug is likely to involve any risk to human beings or animals or that any such drug does not have the therapeutic value claimed, Central Government then in the public interest may prohibit the manufacture, sale or distribution of such drug.

f) Every person, not being the manufacturer of any ASU drug shall disclose to the Inspector; the name, address and other particulars of the person from whom he acquired the ASU drug.

g) Every person holding a license under Section 33-EEC shall keep and maintain such records, registers and other documents as may be prescribed and shall furnish to any officer or authority exercising any power or discharging any function under this Act.

h) Government has the power to make rules in consultation with ASU DTAB regarding the establishments of laboratories for testing purposes, the minimum qualification for analysts and inspectors, methods of analysis, declaring any substance to be poisonous and prescribing Forms for a license for manufacturing ASU drugs.

i) Penalty upon any contravention of the Act shall invite imprisonment upto 1-3 years and/or fine starting from 50,000 to three times the confiscated drug, whichever is more

27. Explain the manufacturing requirements of ASU drugs.

Schedule T of D&C act, 1940 describes the Good Manufacturing Practices for ASU drugs which are described below,

a) **General requirements**: location of the factory involved in the manufacture of ASU drugs should not be in such sites which are close to open drainage, industrial sewage disposal site, drain, public lavatory or any other factories. The building should permit hygienic conditions for manufacturing. Rooms should not be damp and should be well ventilated with adequate fire safety measures. Sufficient measures should be in place for preventing entry of rodents and insects, drying of crude drugs and drainage system.

b) **Water supply**: water used should be pure and of potable quality. Washing of premises by water should be conducted regularly.

c) **Disposal of waste**: waste generated from the manufacturing sections and testing laboratories must be disposed of as per the provisions of pollution control authorities.

d) **Cleaning of containers**: cleaning arrangements for containers used in the manufacturing process must take place in an area separated from the manufacturing area.

e) **Stores**: stores should be well ventilated and free from dampness. Separate storage facility for raw material, packaging material and finished products is required.

f) **Raw materials**: raw materials must be stored in adequate containers as required for preserving the raw material from moisture, rodents and microbial contamination. The containers should be properly labelled, and the current status of the raw material, whether rejected or approved, must be indicated.

   Finished goods stores: the finished goods must be kept in finished goods stores area marked as 'Quarantine'. Only after verification by the quality control team it shall move to approved finished goods stock from where it can be dispatched.

g) **Working space**: the manufacturing area should have proper spacing to allow safe movement and avoid mixing of materials due to space congestion.

h) **Workers**: should be free from any contagious diseases. Proper dressing should be provided, and personal hygiene must be maintained. Adequate medical facilities, including periodic checks ups, must be provided.

i) **Machines and equipment's**: all necessary machines required in the manufacturing must be installed in an orderly manner in a particular manufacturing sequence, ensuring optimal workflow. Standard operating procedures for all equipments must be provided.

j) **Batch manufacturing records**: the licensee must maintain batch manufacturing records for each batch of ASU drugs. Manufacturing records must provide an account of the list of raw materials and their quantities obtained from the store; tests conducted during the various stages of manufacturing.

k) **Distribution Records**: Records of sale and distribution of each batch of ASU Drugs shall be maintained in order to facilitate prompt and complete recall of the batch, if necessary. Records should indicate the date of expiry of the batch. However, formulations like Bhasma, Asava-arishta do not have an expiry date, and their efficacy increases with the passage of time; hence, records must be maintained till 5 years after exhausting the stock.

l) **Record of Market Complaints**: Manufacturers shall maintain a register to record all reports of market complaints received regarding the products sold in the market. The manufacturer shall enter all data received on such market complaints; investigations carried out by the manufacturers regarding the complaint as well as any corrective action initiated to prevent recurrence of such market complaints shall also be recorded.

m) **Quality Control**: Every licensee is required to provide a facility for quality control section on his own premises or through a Government-approved testing laboratory. The tests shall be as per the ASU pharmacopoeia. If specific test protocol is not available, the same shall be performed according to the manufacturers specification or other information available. The quality control section shall verify all the raw materials, monitor in process quality checks and control the quality of the finished product being released.

Brain Teasers (for competitive exams)

1. **Full form of WIPO?**

   World Intellectual Property Organization (WIPO)

2. **Full form of TRIPS**

   Trade related aspects of intellectual property rights, 1995

3. **Criteria of an ideal patent are?**

   Novelty, Non-obviousness and Utility

4. **Tenure of patent is?**

   20 years

5. **In which year Geographical indication of goods act came into existence?**

   1999

6. **Production of new variants of plant species by asexual or transgenic methods is governed by?**

   Plant variety Protection Act

7. **The date on which a patent application is filed for the first time?**

   Priority date

8. **The section of patent office involved in the screening of application?**

   Receipt, Sorting and Distribution (RECS)

9. **In Indian Patent Act, 1970, frivolous inventions come under?**

   Section 3(a)

10. **International agreement for filing patent applications?**

    PCT (Patent Cooperation Treaty)

11. **The first amendment of the Indian Patent act, 1970, was introduced in?**

    1999

12. **Investigation of living things to evaluate how they can be commercially or economically useful to humans is better known as?**

    Bioprospecting or biodiversity prospecting

13. **When traditional knowledge is used for commercialization or patenting without proper authorization or benefit-sharing?**

    Biopiracy

14. **UPOV Stands for?**

    Union for the Protection of New Varieties of Plants

15. **CDSCO Stands for?**

    Central Drug standard Control Organization

16. **For manufacturing Churna and Lepa Ayurvedic formulations, the minimum manufacturing space required is?**

    200 sq ft

17. **Which chapter of D&C Act, 1940 describes the regulation of manufacture and sale of ASU drugs?**

    Chapter IVA

18. **CCRAS stands for**?

Central Council for Research in Ayurveda and Siddha

19. **NMPB stands for?**

National Medicinal Plants Board, Established in 2000

20. **According to which section of D&C Act, 1940, a separate DTAB was constituted for examining ASU drugs?**

33 C

21. **Section 33 D of D&C Act, 1940 describes what type of constitution according to D and C Act 1940?**

Constitution of separate Drug Consultative Committee (SDCC)

22. **Misbranded Drugs?**

Section 33 E

23. **Spurious drugs?**

Section 33EEA

General Introduction of Herbal Industry, Schedule T – GMP of Indian Systems of Medicine

Two marks category questions

1. **Name four herbal drug industriesoperational in India.**
   a) DABUR India Ltd.
   b) Baidyanath
   c) Himalaya
   d) VICCO Laboratories

2. **Name four government institutions engaged in research related to medicinal plants.**
   a) Central Institute of Medicinal and Aromatic Plants (CIMAP)-Lucknow
   b) Central Drug Research Institute (CDRI)- Lucknow
   c) Indian Institute for Integrative Medicines (IIIM)- Jammu
   d) Institute of Himalayan Bioresource Technology, Palampur

3. **Name four societies related to medicinal plant research.**
   a) International Society of Ethnopharmacology
   b) Phytochemical Society of Europe
   c) American Society of Pharmacognosy
   d) Society for Medicinal Plant & Natural Product Research

4. **Name four policy-making agencies in India committed solely to medicinal plant research and regulation.**
   a) The National Medicinal Plants Board
   b) AYUSH
   c) ICMR

5. **Name three autonomous research institutes under DST involved in medicinal plant research.**

   a) Agharkar Research Institute, Pune

   b) Bose Institute, Kolkata

   c) The Institute of Advanced Study in Science & Technology, Guwahati.

6. **Name three government agencies that provides funding for research in medicinal plants.**

   a) National Medicinal Plants Board

   b) Science & Engineering Research Board (SERB)

   c) AYUSH.

7. **Name three indigenously developed herbal medicine by Indian research institutes.**

   a) Anti-diabetic herbal drug BGR-34 which has been developed by two CSIR laboratories - The Central Institute of Medicinal & Aromatic Plants (CIMAP) and the National Botanical Research Institute (NBRI), both located in Lucknow

   b) Standardized extract Dalbergia sissoo developed by CDRI, Lucknow for bone fracture healing

   c) Gugulipid, a hypolipidemic drug developed by CDRI, Lucknow.

8. **Name three journals related to research in medicinal plants.**

   a) Planta Medica

   b) International Journal of Ethnopharmacology

   c) Indian Journal of Experimental Biology.

9. **Define GMP?**

   GMP is that part of Quality Assurance that ensures that products are consistently produced and controlled to the quality standard appropriate to their intended use and as required by the marketing authorization. In simpler words, GMP refers to such practices of production and testing that consistently ensures a quality product. GMP does not provide guidelines on how to manufacture products but provides a series of principles indicating the best practices that must be followed during manufacturing. GMP covers all aspects of the manufacturing process. It provides standard norms regarding suitable premises, storage, transport, quality control personnel, adequate laboratory facilities, approved written procedures and instructions, records to show all steps of defined procedures taken, full traceability of a product through batch processing records and distribution records and systems for recall and investigation of complaints.

10. **What is schedule T?**

Government of India notified 'Schedule T' on 23rd June, 2000 under Rule157 of Drugs & Cosmetic Rules and further amended Good Manufacturing Practices (GMP)

On 07thMarch, 2003. These Rules were made mandatory to all new ASU drug manufacturing units, and already existing ASU manufacturing units were given two years grace period for compliance to Schedule T norms. Schedule T describes the good manufacturing practices for AYUSH drugs. Schedule T specifies the requirements of factory premises and hygienic conditions. The main aim of introducing Schedule-T was to maintain a uniform standard ofhygiene for the manufacturers. Compliance with Good manufacturing Practices as mentioned in Schedule T is mandatory for all the manufacturers of ASU drugs.

11. **What are the objectives of Schedule T under GMP?**

The Good Manufacturing Practices (GMP) are prescribed as follows in Part I and Part II to ensure: -

a) The authenticity of raw materials used in the manufacturing of ASU drugs and to assure their non-contamination status

b) That manufacturing process is according to prescribed norms

c) Adoption of adequate quality control measures

d) That the manufactured drug is of acceptable quality

e) That each licensee shall follow all provisions strictly

f) Adequate documentation during manufacturing.

12. **Name the various national institutes under the AYUSH system established by Central Government.**

a) National Institute of Ayurveda (NIA), Jaipur:

b) Rashtriya Ayurveda Vidyapeeth (RAV), New Delhi

   c) Institute of Post Graduate Teaching and Research in Ayurveda (IPGT&RA), Gujrat

   d) National Institute of Unani Medicine (NIUM), Bengaluru

   e) National Institute of Siddha (NIS), Chennai.

13. Name some medicinal plants which are used mostly for commercial purposes.

Liquorice, Isabgol, Brahmi, Kalmegh, Satavari, Ashwagandha, Chirata, Shankhpushpi, Giloe, *and* Safed Musli.

Five marks category questions

14. Give a brief overview of the Indian herbal drug industries.

Indian herbal market approximately worth near Rs. 50 billion with an annual growth rate of 14%. India exports herbal products worth Rs. 1 billion. According to WHO projections, the global herbal market is likely to grow upto USD 5 trillion by 2050, and India shall be one of the key contributors. India and China are the two biggest countries inAsia in terms of usage of natural resources. According to AYUSH, India ranks as the world's second-largest exporter of medicinal plants after China,according to 2009 data. The Ayurveda market in India was valued at Rs. 300 billion in 2018, and is expected to reach Rs. 710.87 billion by 2024. Rising awareness about the importance of a healthy lifestyle, increasing preference in favour of chemical-free natural products, as well as favourable government ecosystem, have led to the expansion of the herbal market in India. The total amount of herbal raw drugs consumed in India was 319500 metric tons in 2005-2006. Out of this, 17000 metric tons was used by herbal drug industries. In 2010, about 1650 herbal formulations were available in the Indian market, reflecting the huge volume of herbal drug industries. Nearly 8000 medicinal plants are currently used by the herbal industries. Presently, the United States is the largest market for Indian botanical products accounting for about 50% of the exports. The major herbals exported from India in recent years are isabgol, opium alkaloids, senna derivatives, vinca extract, cinchona alkaloids, menthol, gymnema herb etc. There are more than 8000 herbal drug manufacturers in India. Major players operating in the Indian herbal products market include Dabur India Limited, Emami Limited, Patanjali Ayurveda Limited, The Himalaya Drug Company, Sandu Pharmaceuticals Limited, and Shahnaz Ayurveda Private Limited. Baidyanath, Dabur, and Emami together account for about 85% share of the country's herbal market.

15. **Explain the challenges associated with the herbal drug industry.**

   a) Challenges related to regulatory issues: herbal medicines are often released into the market without performing mandatory safety or toxicological investigations. Very few countries have an effective system to regulate manufacturing practices and quality standards of herbal medicine. Challenges are faced regarding satisfying regulatory agencies on issues pertaining to the assessment of safety, efficacy and quality control of herbal medicines. The lack of pharmacovigilance data on herbal medicines is also worsening the situation further.

   b) Assessment of safety and efficacy: since a single herbal drug contains various phytoconstituents, it becomes difficult to develop an assay procedure for all constituents present in the crude drug. The situation becomes further complicated in the case of polyherbal formulations, which contains multiple crude drugs.

   c) Quality control of herbal medicines: the following are a matter of concern for the herbal drug industries,

   • Quality of herbal raw material

   • Correct identification of the plant species

   • GMP compliance

   • Heavy metal contamination

   • Pesticide residues

   d) Safety monitoring of herbal medicines: pharmacovigilance and communication of such data to the regulatory authorities and cooperation between physicians and traditional practioners are needed to identify early signs of any adverse reactions or herb-drug interactions. Independent scientific investigation like toxicological, evaluation and botanical verification can be a valuable addition.

e) Capacity building in cultivation and harvesting:

- Over exploitation to be avoided
- Destructive harvesting can affect local biodiversity leading to the non-availability of crude drugs
- Controlled use of pesticides and insecticides.

16. Explain the future prospects of the herbal drug industry.

i. Awareness in using medicinal plants among urban and city people

ii. Promotion of ethnobotanical exploration

iii. Adequate quality assurance protocol for herbal medicines to eliminate adulteration

iv. Production, sale and use of herbal medicine should be controlled through well-framed legislations

v. Integration of modern medicine with traditional knowledge in a holistic way

vi. Isolation, identification of pure bioactive compounds and their subsequent chemical synthesis to ensure a sustainable supply of such bioactive compounds

vii. Cultivation of commercially important medicinal plants in wasteland areas

viii. Generate new jobs through realistic policies with the economic outlook

ix. Conservation of biodiversity and prevention of bio-piracy

x. Developing ecosystem which supports socio-economic growth.

17. Mention the principles of GMP.

a) Manufacturing processes are clearly defined, controlled and validated to ensure consistency and compliance with specifications.

b) Any changes to the approved process are documented and evaluated. Changes that have an impact on the quality of the drug are validated as necessary.

c) Instructions and procedures are written in clear and unambiguous language.

d) Operators are trained to carry out and document procedures.

e) Records are maintained throughout the manufacturing process, and detailed notes for each manufacturing step are documented. Deviations are investigated and documented. Records of manufacture (including distribution) that enable the complete history of a batch to be traced are retained in a comprehensible and accessible form.

f) A system is kept in place for recalling any batch of drug from sale or supply if the need for so arises.

g) Complaints about marketed drugs are examined, causes of quality defects are investigated, and appropriate measures are taken with respect to the defective drugs so that their occurrence can be prevented in the future.

18. List out the different components of GMP.

GMP has two components, PART I &PART II.

Part I:

Good manufacturing practices for premises and materials,

1)   General requirements
   a) Location and surroundings
   b) Building and premises
   c) Water system
   d) Disposal of waste
2)   Warehousing area
3)   Production area
4)   Ancillary areas
5)   Quality control area
6)   Personnel
7)   Health, clothing and sanitation of workers
8)   Manufacturing operations & controls
9)   Sanitation in manufacturing premises
10) Raw materials
11) EQUIPMENT

12) Documentation and records

13) Labels and other printed materials

14) Quality assurance

15) Self-inspection and Quality audit

16) Master formula records

17) Packaging records

18) Batch processing records

19) Standard operating procedures (SOP)

20) Reference samples

21) Reprocessing and recording

22) Distribution records

23) Product recalls

24) Complaints and adverse reactions

25) Site master file

Part II:

Requirements of Plant and Equipment

19. **Explain the provisions related to working space under Schedule T for the manufacturing of ASU drugs.**

Working space:

a) Location of rest and refreshment rooms shall be totally separate from manufacturing and quality control areas

b) Facilities for changing and storing clothes and for washing/toilet purposes should be easily accessible and appropriate for the number of users. Toilets shall not provide direct passage to production or storage areas.

c) Spare parts and tools should be stored in the production area under lock and key.

d) Animal houses should be well isolated from other areas, with separate entrances.

e) The manufacturing area should provide adequate space for orderly placement of Equipment's and other material so as to avoid congestion and provide easy and safe working without any possibility of mixing of raw materials or products or any cross-contamination.

20. **Explain the norms of storage area under Schedule T for the manufacturing of ASU drugs.**

Storage area:

a) Storage areas should have sufficient capacity to allow orderly storage of the various categories of materials and products with proper separation and segregation. Starting and packaging materials, intermediates, bulk and finished products, products in quarantine, and released, rejected, returned, or recalled products must be stored separately.

b) Storage areas should be designed to ensure good storage conditions in terms of illumination, ventilation, cleanliness, temperature and humidity. Special storage conditions required for certain herbal materials and finished preparations should be provided if required, with proper documentation.

c) Separate receiving and dispatch points shall be made in the storage area. Receiving areas should facilitate the cleaning of containers of incoming materials if so required.

d) Quarantine areas must be designated inside the storage section for the storage of finished products before going out for commercial distribution. Such areas should be well labelled and properly demarcated, and their access restricted to authorized personnel only.

e) Proper segregation should be provided for the storage of rejected, recalled, or returned materials or products.

f) Radioactive materials, narcotics and other dangerous drugs, and substances capable of causing biohazard, risks of abuse upon consumption, fire or explosion should be stored in safe and secure areas.

g) Printed packaging materials are critical to the conformity and establishing the identity of any pharmaceutical product. Hence such materials must be securely stored.

h) Sampling activity in storage must not lead to cross-contamination.

21. **Explain the requirements of machinery and equipments under Schedule T for the manufacturing of ASU drugs.**

Machinery & equipment's:

A. Equipment must be located, designed, constructed, and maintained as per the operations to be carried out in the manufacturing unit. Equipment's must be cleaned and maintained effectively to avoid cross-contamination, build-up of dust or dirt so that there is no adverse effect on the quality of products.

B. There should be adequate space between machines for the orderly movement of personnel and ease of operations.

C. Proper standard operational procedures (SOPs) for cleaning, maintaining and calibrating every machine should be prescribed.

D. The fixed pipeline should be clearly labelled to indicate the contents and direction of flow.

E. All service piping and devices should be adequately marked, and special attention should be paid to the non-interchangeable connections or adaptors for the presence of any dangerous gases and liquids.

F. Balances and other measuring equipments of an appropriate range and precision should be available for production and control operations and should be calibrated on a regular basis.

G. Washing, cleaning and drying of equipment should be done so that such equipment's or containers does not become a source of contamination.

H. Production equipment should not present any hazard to the products. The parts of the production equipment that come into contact with the product shall not be reactive, additive, or absorptive to the extent that would affect the quality of the product. Nonwooden equipment should be used unless tradition demands wooden material. When wooden equipment is used, it is advisable that it does not come into direct contact with chemicals.

I. Defective eqipments's should be removed from production and quality control areas or else clearly labelled as defective to prevent use.

J. Closed equipment's should be used whenever appropriate. Where open equipment is used, precautions shall be taken to minimize contamination.

K. Vacuum or wet-cleaning methods are preferred. If wet-cleaning is done, the equipment should be dried immediately after cleaning to prevent the growth of microorganisms.

L. Current drawings of critical equipment's and support systems should be maintained.

22. **Explain standard operating procedures mentioned under Schedule T for the manufacturing of ASU drugs.**

Standard operating procedures:

a) Standard operating procedures and associated records should be available for equipment assembly and validation, analytical apparatus, maintenance, cleaning and sanitization, personnel matters including qualification, training, clothing, pest control, complaints, recalls, returns, handling of hazardous materials, entry and exit from production areas etc.

b) There should be SOP's and records for the receipt of each delivery of starting material and printed packaging material.

c) There should be SOP's for internal labelling, quarantine and storage of starting materials, packaging materials and other materials, as appropriate.

d) SOP's for sampling which should specify the person(s) authorized to take samples.

e) SOP's describe the details of the batch number, with the intention of ensuring that each batch of intermediate, bulk or finished product is identified with a specific batch number.

f) There should be written procedures for testing materials and products at different stages of manufacturing, describing the methods and equipment's to be used.

g) Written release and rejection procedures should be available for materials and products.

h) SOP's describe responsibilities for cleaning and sanitation with details regarding cleaning schedules, methods, equipment, and materials to be used and facilities and equipment's to be cleaned.

23. **Explain the provisions associated with the health and hygiene of factory workers under Schedule T for the manufacturing of ASU drugs.**

Health & hygiene:

a) All personnel, before being appointed for the job and during their working, shall undergo health examinations as specified.

Personnel conducting visual inspections shall also undergo periodic eye examinations.

b) All personnel shall undergo mandatory training on good hygienic practices to be followed. Signs and posters giving visual instructions for maintaining hygiene must be displayed at appropriate places.

c) Any person showing symptoms of any illness or open lesions that may adversely affect the quality of products shall not be allowed to handle the manufacturing process and finished goods.

d) All employees should be instructed to immediately report about their health issues if any.

e) There shall be no direct contact between the bare hands of personnel's and starting materials, primary packaging materials and intermediate or bulk products.

f) To ensure self-protection and avoid product contamination, personnel must wear all protective and manufacturing clothing as required.

g) Smoking, eating, drinking, chewing, and keeping plants, food, drink, personal medicines, incense sticks, garlands etc., shall be permitted only in designated places and strictly not inside the production, laboratory or storage area.

Ten marks category questions

24. **Explain in detail the infrastructural requirements under Schedule T for the manufacturing of ASU drugs.**

Infrastructural requirements:

a) Premises must be located, designed, constructed, adapted, and maintained to suit the operations to be carried out as required for the manufacturing of ASU drugs.

b) The layout and design of premises shall be such that it minimizes the risk of errors, permits effective cleaning and maintenance to avoid cross-contamination. Accumulation of dust or dirt should be avoided (walls should not be damp and should be free from cracks and the floor should be smooth and even in nature).

c) Operations like sampling, mixing, powder packaging etc., which are likely to generate dust, measures shall be taken to avoid cross-contamination through adequate cleaning and ventilation.

d) Premises should be situated in an environment where chances of contamination of product are at the minimum.

e) Premises must maintain good sanitation, adequate fire safety measures and enough exits in case of an emergency.

f) Premises shall be carefully maintained, and it shall be ensured that repair and maintenance operations do not present any hazard to the quality of products.

g) Premises shall be cleaned and disinfected regularly.

h) Electrical supply, lighting, temperature, humidity and ventilation shall be appropriate and such that they do not adversely affect AYUSH products, either at the manufacturing stage or during storage, or even the accurate functioning of equipment's.

i) Premises should be designed and equipped so as to prevent the entry of insects, birds or animals. There shall be a procedure for rodent and pest control.

j) Premises shall be designed to ensure the logical flow of materials and personnel.

25. **Explain what kind of documentation and record-keeping is required under Schedule T for the manufacturing of ASU drugs.**

Documentation:

a) All documents should be approved, signed and dated by the competent authority. Changes to any document should be done only post-authorization.

b) Documents should not have confusing and misleading contents, and all information with title, nature and purpose should be clearly stated.

c) Documents should be regularly reviewed and kept up to date.

d) Documentation should be completed immediately after the completion of the action; documentation should be such that all manufacturing events of a particular batch are traceable.

e) Records should be retained for at least one year after the expiry date of the finished product.

Records

Batch processing records:

a) A batch processing record shall be kept for each batch processed.

b) Proper records regarding the equipment's/work station, its cleaning status and confirmation of making the instrument free from any contamination must be documented before the starting of a fresh batch.

c) During processing, information such as the name of the product, number of the batch, dates and time of commencement of production, name of the person responsible, name of the operator, in-process controls performed, amount of product obtained, and any special observation shall be recorded during each production. Such documents shall be duly signed by the competent authority.

Batch packaging records:

a) Batch packaging records shall be preserved for each batch or part batch processed.

b) Records must indicate that before beginning any packaging operations, the equipment was thoroughly cleaned, and all traces of previous batch products which could serve as contaminants has been removed.

c) The following information such as the name of the product, batch number and quantity, date and time of the packaging operations, name of in-charge, initials of the operators, checks made for identity and conformity with the packaging instructions, details of the packaging operations carried out, quantities and reference number or identification of all printed packaging materials and bulk product issued, used, destroyed or returned to stock, all such information shall be recorded each time along with the date and the person responsible should be clearly identified by signature or electronic password.

Brain Teasers (for competitive exams)

1. **NBRI stands for**

   National Botanical Research Institute, UP

2. **Central Institute of Medicinal and Aromatic Plants is located in which city?**

   Lucknow (UP)

3. **When was Central Drug Research Institute (CDRI) inaugurated?**

   17th Feb 1951

4. **NBPGR stands for?**

   National Bureau of Plant Genetic Resources

5. **Dabur India Ltd was established in?**

   1884 (Dr.S.K.Burman Founder of Dabur India Ltd.)

6. **Odonil is used as?**

   Air fresheners

7. **BaidyanathAyurved company was established in?**

   1917 by Pt Ram Dayal Joshi

8. **Himalaya Drug company was established by?**

   M. Manal in 1930 based in Bangalore

9. **Liv-52 is flagship herbal product of?**

   Himalaya Drug Company, launched in 1955 used as Hepatoprotective

10. **Natural Remedies Pvt. Ltd. was founded by?**

    R. K. Agrawal in 1951 (Bangalore)

11. **Vajradanti is the flagship product of?**

    Vicco Laboratories Pvt Ltd

12. **Navratna Cool oil is a flagship product of?**

    Emami Group

13. **Herbokam (Anti-stress formula) is a proprietary product of?**

Universal/Unijules Medicaments

14. **Patanjali Ayurved was launched in?**

2006

15. **Nutrilite is a product of?**

Amway

16. **Certificate of renewal for carrying out tests or analysis on ASU drugs or raw materials used in manufacture thereof on behalf of the licensee for manufacture for sale of ASU drugs.**

Form 49

17. **Approval for carrying out tests or analysis on ASU drugs or raw materials used in manufacture thereof on behalf of licensee s for manufacture for sale of ASU drugs.**

Form 48

18. **In the Unani system of medicine, Nasal drops are better known as?**

Saoot

19. **According to the Ayurvedic system of medicine, Swarsasa relates to?**

Fresh juice

20. **Certificate of Good Manufacturing Practices (GMP) to Manufacturer of ASU Drugs?**

Form 26E-I

21. **Certificate of renewal of loan license to manufacture for sale of ASU drugs?**

Form 26-E

www.ingramcontent.com/pod-product-compliance
Lightning Source LLC
Chambersburg PA
CBHW050754150726

48196CB00004B/469